EMPOWERED FOR CHANGE TO ACHIEVE TOTAL WELL-BEING

You have what it takes

Cecily Mwaniki

authorHOUSE®

AuthorHouse™ UK Ltd.
500 Avebury Boulevard
Central Milton Keynes, MK9 2BE
www.authorhouse.co.uk
Phone: 08001974150

First published by AuthorHouse 03/12/2011

ISBN: 978-1-4567-7547-6(sc)
ISBN: 978-1-4567-7548-3 (e)

The paradox of our time in history is that we have taller buildings but shorter tempers, wider freeways, but narrower viewpoints. We spend more, but have less; we buy more, but enjoy less. We have bigger houses and smaller families, more conveniences, but less time. We have more degrees but less sense, more knowledge, but less judgment, more experts, yet more problems, more medicine, but less wellness.

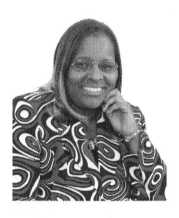

(George Carlin, comedian of the 70s and 80s)

He who is not aware of his ignorance will only be misled by his knowledge. I cannot only use all the brains that I have, but all that I can borrow. Hard work never killed anybody and bear in mind that procrastination is the thief of time. Start every day with a smile and get it over with.

(Richard Whatley)

Dedication

I dedicate this book to my family, whom I love to see fulfill their potential on this planet earth. I broaden this dedication to include all those who boldly dare to adjust for the most desired change in their lives. As one woman who faces changes and even disappointments, I want to encourage you: never give up; never give in; and for God's sake, never give out! I believe the best is yet to come. I further broaden this dedication with love to include all the families of yesterday, today, and tomorrow – may we always support one another and wish each other health and wealth.

Acknowledgements

My parents: To say, as I have always maintained, that you are my role models, my inspiration, my life coaches and mentors – though true – seems shallow and ineffective in communicating who you are and your great meaning in my life.

I extend my sincere gratitude to my family, who shared me with this manuscript. I will always appreciate your love, companionship, and support.

I also want to acknowledge the companionship and encouragement that I constantly received, in one way or another, from all those involved in the Utulivu organization. You have remained the basis of my social, spiritual, and even intellectual growth. The inspiration, encouragement, and challenges I get from the work of Utulivu are incredible.

Feasts of literature and lengthy interactions with great minds have not cured my malady of expression.

What you leave behind is not what is engraved in the stone monuments but what is woven into the lives of others.

(Greek politician)

CONTENTS

INTRODUCTION

As I write this, the cold season has already set in. It has been worse in the last couple of days, and the weather forecast continues to warn for the worst. The last thing anyone wants to do, therefore, is to go out in the chill and the snow. This is not a one-day inconvenience; it is going to be like this for several weeks. I don't like it. The worst is that I am aware I cannot change it. One day last year, it actually snowed so much that I was stuck on the road from work for six and a half hours instead of the usual fifteen minutes it takes me to get home. It was the same the year before and as far back as you want to go. Barring climatic changes, it's going to happen again next year and for many years to come. That is the reality of the seasons. We do not determine them.

This leaves me with two options. I could sit all day and complain about the foul weather, take a break for my sleep tonight, and resume my complaining tomorrow morning. On the other hand, I could dress warmly, make myself a flask of hot chocolate, and catch up with my writing and other things that need to be done. That way, this terrible weather would turn into an opportunity.

Just as the earth goes through climatic seasons, our lives, too, must go through inescapable seasons. Of course, we enjoy the warmth of the "springs" and "summers" of our lives, when everything falls into place. Unfortunately, we wrongly assume that this should be all there is to our lives. This is not reality. If there is a summer, there is going to be a winter, with springs and autumns providing the bridges between the two.

As a mother of two girls, I have had opportunity to watch my kids respond to the changing seasons of their lives. I must admit that they do a better job of responding to the seasons than adults do. For a first example, I never taught any of them to suckle. Once they came out of the womb, they instinctively knew the season had changed. They knew dinner time was going to take another shape. All they needed was to be put next to my breast. Not only did they know what to do, but they did it with all their strength. However, if I forgot to do what I needed to do, they would holler until I did!

Then came the time when they knew they needed to transport themselves from one place to another. Without an instructor, they began to crawl. Then they learnt to walk, to run, and so forth. Somehow, along the way, they noticed that other people had a better way of communicating than by crying. So they began to talk. At some point afterwards, they noticed that other people went to school. They immediately began to desire school and demand to be enrolled.

None of these seasons was easy for them. Each presented its own challenges – and sometimes even a measure of trauma. My little ones could not be tucked back. Each season presented a measure of frustration, failure, and even pain. But they always got up and tried again, and in the end, they conquered each season

As children, we all go through those victories. However, something goes wrong once we enter adulthood. We stop anticipating the seasons. Everything seems to take us off-guard, leaving us murmuring with discontent. The sad result is that our lives end up being a catalogue of missed opportunities and a source of discontent. How sad!

As long as we are on earth, we have no option but to expect and accept the reality of the seasons. As we all know, some seasons are more desirable than others. We cannot, however, choose to have one season and not the others. Every season will come upon us whether we like it or not. The only thing left to us is to decide how the seasons will affect us. Our immediate task is to make sure that we control how the seasons affect us, because what we do not control will control us. The goal should be that no season should leave us the way it found us. We have to change; if we don't, it means we did not embrace the season and make it work for us. The secret is that once we know the season, we must allow ourselves to experience it. We must not cushion ourselves from what God is doing in our lives at that time, even if it is painful. Above all, we must do more than just accept the season. We must appreciate it as a good thing, as a vital ingredient in God's plan. We must be prepared to adapt to new challenges and develop endurance to face life's unending battles. I tried to describe what life is to my daughter Mercy in my first book, *Becoming the Better You*. Here's what I told her:

- Life is a challenge; meet it.
- Life is a gift; accept it.

- Life is an adventure; overcome it.

- Life is a tragedy; face it.

- Life is a duty; perform it.

- Life is a song; sing it.

- Life is an opportunity; take it.

- Life is a journey; complete it.

- Life is beauty; praise it.

- Life is a struggle; fight it.

- Life is a goal; achieve it.

- Life is a puzzle; solve it.

Be wise, therefore; live it well and celebrate it. Above all, seek God's wisdom in order to recognize the season you are in, as this will empower you for change in all aspects of your life. You will thereby achieve man's most-needed goal of total well-being for a healthier and wealthier family. This will no doubt lead to a healthier and wealthier society, as God intends it to be.

CHAPTER 1:

CHANGE TO ACHIEVE

A winner never quits, and a quitter never wins: Everything starts with a beginning. Nobody can go back and start a new beginning, but anyone can start today and make a new ending. Remember, in everything, your altitude determines your aptitude.

Unknown

Where Does Change Begin?

Everything big starts with something small, and nothing great is created suddenly. Everything can be done little by little; therefore, never decide to do nothing just because you can only do something small. Within a little thing lies a big opportunity; small things make a difference. Therefore, do all that it takes to be successful in little things. Personally, I always ask God to send me small opportunities in my life, because I know that if I am faithful in the small things, bigger opportunities will open up to me. One of the major differences between people who have momentum and those who don't is that those with momentum are growing by taking advantage of small opportunities. In most cases, the impossible is the untried. I therefore encourage you to do something; adjust yourself for change. The courage to begin is the same courage it takes to succeed. This is the courage that separates dreamers from achievers. The beginning is the most important part of any endeavor. Worse than a quitter is someone who is afraid to begin. Ninety per cent of success is showing up and starting. You may be disappointed if you fail, but you are doomed if you don't try. Remember, simply knowing where you want to go cannot be a substitute for putting one foot in front of the other. People, like trees, must grow or wither – there is no standing still. Therefore, dare to *begin*!

Change, but Don't Stop

When you are through changing, you are through with life. Many people fail in life because they are unwilling to make changes, and therefore, they decide to quit. The fact is that correction and change always bear fruit. All humankind is divided into three classes: those who are unchangeable, those who are changeable, and those who cause change.

Change is always hardest for the man who is in a rut. This is because he has scaled down his living to that which he can handle comfortably, and he welcomes no change or challenge that would lift him up.

If you find yourself in a hole, stop digging. When things go wrong, don't go with them. Stubbornness and unwillingness to change represent the energy of fools. Sir Francis Bacon wrote "He that will not apply new remedies must expect new evils."

In the Bible, Psalm 32:8, we are reassured that the Lord will instruct us and guide us along the best pathways for our lives; He will advise us and watch our progress.

God never closes one door without opening another one. We must be willing to change in order to walk through a new door. In prayer, we learn to change, so we can walk through that new door. Prayer is one of the most life-altering experiences we will ever know. We cannot pray and stay the same.

Playing it safe is probably the most unsafe thing in the world. We cannot stand still. We must go forward and be open to those adjustments that God has for us. The unhappy are those who fear change. We cannot make omelettes without breaking eggs. Accomplishment automatically results in change. One change makes way for the next, giving us the opportunity to grow. We must continue to change in order to master change.

We must be open to change – because every time we think we are ready to graduate from the school of experience, somebody thinks up a new course. We must consciously be willing to experience change. If we can figure when to stand firm and when to bend, we've got it made. We need to welcome change as a friend. We can become nervous because of incessant change, but we would be frightened if the change were stopped.

Blessed is the man who can adjust to a state of circumstances without surrendering his convictions. We must open our arms to change but not let go of our values. People often meet with failure because they don't persist in developing new ideas or make plans to take the place of those that failed. Our growth depends on our willingness to experience change.

If God simply handed us everything we wanted, He would be taking from us our greatest prize – the joy of accomplishment.

Never Settle for Less

If you grew up not knowing love; if your parents were always fighting, and all you knew was hatred, anger, and animosity, your response to love would be affected by this experience. Whatever you saw and experienced as you grew up would continue to inform your beliefs. You would grow up believing that women should be beaten, because that is what you grew up seeing, and it's now programmed in your mind. Since you grew up not receiving the kind of love that God intended for you, you would treat with suspicion any overtures of love. Your upbringing has developed into a belief system, and then it translated into a response. This response has crystallized into an experience – a continuous, unchanging reality.

Imagination is an inbuilt compass or radar that God intended to lead you to your future. Any negative circumstance that happens in your imagination becomes a limitation. Once your imagination is limited, your future is limited. When your vision of what you are expecting to become is limited, your future is limited.

To raise the standard, your mind must be in agreement with your aspirations. It must see the possibility of what you are aspiring towards. It may be necessary to allow your mind to be deprogrammed and then reprogrammed. That will involve letting go of the lies that have kept you captive and accepting God's redeeming truths. Before you can be filled, you have to be emptied. God cannot fill you unless you are empty. So empty yourself of every negative experience and memory from the past; empty yourself of every downfall and of every curse. Empty yourself of everything you cannot be, and let God fill you with who He calls you to be. Emptying yourself is not easy, but it is not a choice. If you have grown up being called stupid, you must come to that place where you are able to say "I am not stupid." I might have grown up being told I'm not beautiful, but I *am* beautiful. What does the Word say? You are what the Word says you are. You are who God says you are. You are fearfully and wonderfully made. You were cut out for a purpose and called to make a difference in this life. Don't settle for less!

Put Your Energy to Better Use

It is far better to use your energy to change the things you don't like, but you won't if you spend your life listening to the "knockers". Like poison, their views will affect the way you think. Instead of thinking that all things are possible, you will be telling yourself that things are too hard. You will have given up even before you have dipped a toe into the water and tried something new. I understand how tempting it is to join the knocking brigade. It is a chance to air your views, and even be a bit clever, without actually having to do anything else. And it is a way of telling yourself you are above it all and that you could do things if you wanted to, but you have chosen not to. We are all guilty of this, but if you do it on a regular basis, then you will eventually find it very hard to make changes in your life. To be able to make these changes, you need a more positive outlook. So, to make a start, you must control the negative thoughts you have about others. I am not saying you should not have a friendly little moan with your mates on a Saturday evening or over the phone. What I am saying is, don't turn it into a lifetime habit. It is a well-known fact that knockers have never changed anything worth changing.

It is a fact that people don't like facing up to change. Knockers come in some unexpected disguises. Sometimes even the people closest to you will make it difficult for you to succeed. Have you ever told your family and friends your latest plans and found their response lukewarm? You tell them you plan to spend a year overseas, but instead of being excited for you, they point out the problems they are sure you are going to have. You will be alone, they say; you will not make friends; you don't speak the language; what if you are robbed – or even worse? Don't be surprised by all this. It is likely that they just do not understand what you are doing and therefore find it hard to support you. Most people fear change; if somebody close to them makes a move, it forces them to think about their own lives when they don't want to. The story of the overweight woman who wants to slim down but is told by her friends, "Oh, you don't need to; we love you exactly as you are" shows the sneaky tactics people will use to keep someone where she is. The reason they don't want her to lose weight is that it will change her as a person, and it may very well change the friendship. To stop that happening, her friends try to scupper her efforts. They are not nasty people, but they are afraid.

To prevent people from destroying your efforts, you need to find sources of genuine support. You can do this by making sure you spend more time with people who want you to succeed and be happy in your life. Do not hang around with people who want to throw you off your success, no matter how well-meaning they are. I am not talking about people who offer intelligent, thoughtful views and ideas – always welcome them in your life; however, refuse to be with people who always point out the problems. This is because, if you listen to the knockers, you will never start anything worthwhile. Note that knockers have never changed anything worth changing – they know the value of nothing and are not very good on the price. The thought that you might fail should not stop you making an effort. If you do fail, at least you tried. Above all, make the change you want to see. Stop complaining about what does not work. Do something other than blow hot air at everybody else.

Cecily Mwaniki

Look at yourself first before you judge others. *For every negative thought about someone else's actions, try to think how you would have done it better – that way you will end up a positive being.*

How Much Childhood Have You Retained In Your Adulthood?

Belief, hope, faith, innocence, and sharing of actions are all ingredients that make up the simplicity of being a child. If I had to define *youth*, it would be with those words. Why do I choose those particular words?

Children *believe* in life, while adults refuse to believe in the unknown. Adults have to be given facts, figures, statistics, logic, and existence. If it can happen, an adult has to dissect it to the core to find out the reasons why, how, what, where, and when. We insist on obtainable results that are favorable to our professional and personal lives.

Children believe in *hope* of life, the magical, unseen element of human feel-good that eyes cannot visually portray but the mind feels – the good vibes of hope. Where do adults lose that hope in their journey? What circumstances affect an adult to make him forget the simple joy of invisible hope? It is a lost childhood trait, which allows a child to be friends with anyone, no matter what their gender or race and with no fear of persecution or public humiliation. Adults limit their lives and lifestyles, because they lose hope in themselves and others.

Faith is child's best protector and guidance in life. A child can take the worst circumstance and change the bad to make it good. Faith is a gift that adults tend to abuse. It is the forgotten state of mind that says *yes* – all people are worth the effort. Free and good intentions do still live on. Faith does not ever give up, unless we choose to allow our circumstances to cause it. Faith is creating a dream and following it through. It is grabbing the hand of a best friend and sharing the greatest adventures possible to light up memories for him and those around him.

Innocence does not provoke fear in a child. Innocence will not abuse a child. Innocence is a gift that all adult humans have, if they are only willing to reach deep enough into their souls to touch the truth of their lives. Innocence never leaves anyone, but circumstances will make us believe otherwise, and adults will lie about it.

My favorite, which children do so proudly, is *sharing with actions*. Children have no hidden motive when they communicate with one another or when they find things to occupy their time. Children will share through their actions, and within two seconds, they will fight and make up or hug and laugh. Adults carry ice cubes in their pockets when they have been wronged. They never forget. Children forgive and continue to go on sharing their actions. Why can't adults do this?

As adult parents or guardians, in our professional and personal lives, we have more to learn about ourselves and the contributions that we really give back to others in these lessons from children. It is not our biological ages, or our educational and professional accomplishments, or even public notoriety that make us somebody special – or even qualify us to call ourselves adults.

Honesty, the way I view adults, are in these very elements of a child. I do believe when I should not. I do hope in others when they give me no reason to. I do have faith in a mustard seed (Matthew 17: 20); I believe that if you dream and are willing to work for what you want, dreams do come true. I do see the innocence in the best and worst of all human beings, but I can't make anyone believe this about themselves. Most importantly, I believe that sharing through actions will create and move miracles of humanity when there seems to be no logical, statistical, or rational way to do it. It is for this reason that the childishness in your adulthood will determine how much you are willing to change in order to meet your most desired goals in life.

Never Surrender Your Dreams to Noisy Negatives

Nobody can ever make you feel average without your permission. Ingratitude and criticism are going to come; they are part of the price you pay for leaping past mediocrity.

Learn to expect ingratitude and criticism, because the only way to avoid them is to do nothing and, of course, do nothing. Those who do things inevitably stir up criticism. Did you know that a critic is a man who knows the way but can't drive the car? We should never judge people by what their enemies say about them. Often, criticism will present the best platform from which to proclaim the truth. The good news is that we are not called to respond to criticism but to God. In most cases, people who are critical are either envious or uninformed. They usually say things that have no impact whatsoever upon the truth. There is an anonymous saying that describes this situation perfectly: "It is useless for the sheep to pass resolutions in favour of vegetarianism while the wolf remains of a different opinion."

If what you do and say is of good and of God, it will not make any difference if every other person on the face of the earth criticizes you. Likewise, if what you are doing is not of God, nothing other people say will make it right. So by all means, pay no attention to negative criticism. Trust in the Lord, and do good knowing that in the end what you do in the Lord will be rewarded. Learn to be a blessing to another person and understand that the real art of conversation is not only to say the right thing in the right place but to leave unsaid the wrong thing at tempting moments.

It is important to note that courage is not a lack of fear but the ability to act while facing fear. Remember that the best way to predict your future is to create it. People may doubt what you say, but they will believe what you do. Therefore, be nice to people on your way up, because you will need them on your way down. Never explain; your friends do not need it, and your enemies will not believe it. Always ask God to remind you that His love is greater than your disappointments and His plans are always better than your dreams. Bear in mind that smooth roads hardly make good drivers; clear skies never make good pilots; and calm seas never make good sailors. Similarly, a problem-free life never makes a strong person. Be strong enough, therefore, to accept the challenges of life, and avoid asking "Why me?" Instead say, "With God by my side, *try* me." It is a fact that the enemy never fights a retreating battle, but rather an advancing one, so when you face opposition, press on, knowing that you are going in the right direction. Every day, die in self-ego, and don't give up. Don't quit, but keep pressing on, because you are a winner. Always give a thousand chances to your enemy to become your friend, but don't give a single chance to your friend to become your enemy.

Avoid putting yourself down while looking at the fashions out there. Instead, walk out into the fields and look at the wildflowers. They never primp or shop, but have you ever seen colour and design quite like it? If God gives such attention to the appearance of the wildflowers, don't you think He will attend to you, take pride in you, and do His best for you?

Ignore negative attitudes from those dearest and nearest to you. If you want to change, you must be ready to accept criticism; otherwise, you will not be taking your position. People will talk about your past when you try to occupy your space/position. You may not have what your friends have, but you may have what he does not have. You may not be where you want to be, but you are not where you used to be. You therefore owe God gratitude. Be extraordinary by making yourself above average. Believe in yourself.

Don't just focus on where you are today – envision where you want to be next year. Remember that your today is 100 per cent the fruit of all the wise and not-so-wise decisions you made last year. Also, you don't have to be great to get started, but to become great, you must get started. As you do so, be humble. Avoid raising your status through lowering others' self-esteem.

How Has Recession Changed You?

Has recession broken your nine-to-five grind? According to a report by leading think tank NEF (New Economics Foundation), the recession has led to increasing numbers of people in the United Kingdom working shorter hours, and the trend is set to continue. The company sees this as a positive opportunity for UK PLC. Anna Coute, head of social policy, says, "So many of us live to work, work to earn, and earn to consume." It is unfortunate that our consumption habits are squandering the earth's natural resources. Spending less time in paid work could help us break this pattern. We would have more time to be better parents, better citizens, better carers, and better neighbours. We could also become better employees, less stressed, more in control, happier in our jobs, and more productive. It is time to break the power of the old industrial clock, take back our lives, and work for a sustainable future.

Strategies for Success

Success in life is not achieved by luck or chance but rather by choice. It takes a lot of hard work and dedication. A lot of people want to be successful, and that is why they are full of dreams for the future; however, if you ask them whether they can fulfill those dreams, they don't think they can. Do not think for a moment that you need a master's degree to achieve fulfilment. Just understand that you must have sufficient education, ample experience, or proper training to develop the wisdom that serves as a rung on your ladder to success. Too many people think it is a matter of luck. However, it is important to note that luck can be defined as preparation meeting opportunity.

I wish to share with you something that a good friend emailed me. It made me realize that the most important strategies for success are already within my reach. I already possess them – the task for me is only to put them into action. The email went as follows:

When I woke up this morning, lying in bed, I was asking myself: What are some of the secrets of success in life? I found the answer right there, in my room:

The fan said: Be cool.

The roof said: Aim high.

The window said: See the world.

The clock said: Every minute is precious.

The mirror said: Reflect before you act.

The calendar said: Be up to date.

The door said: Push hard for your goal.

And, not to be forgotten, the carpet said: Kneel down and pray.

Always carry the heart that never hates, a smile that never fades, a touch that never hurts, and above all, have a purposeful day by aiming to be a blessing to others.

This message greatly challenged me to accept the fact that success is already within me. I only need to realize it and use it to make the world a better place.

CHAPTER 2:

MANHOOD AND WOMANHOOD: EFFECTS ON THE IDEAL FAMILY WELL-BEING

By wisdom a house is built, and by understanding it is established; by knowledge the rooms are filled with all precious and pleasant riches (Proverbs 24:3). Marriage, through which a family is established, is an exclusive union between one man and one woman, publicly acknowledged, permanently sealed, and physically consummated.

(Author Nancy Van Pelt)

There are three major stages of life in human beings. These are birth, marriage, and death. All three are important stages, and man strives to go through them gracefully. Marriage marks the climax of the three stages – it is ideally the most fascinating stage in life. Practically, however, this is not always the case, and this adversely affects the total well-being of man. He is therefore not achieving the healthy and wealthy life he desires for his family and the society. The question is, why is this? Read on, and decide whether womanhood and manhood have anything to do with this dilemma.

Fascinating Womanhood

Apply *fascinating womanhood* with restraint at first, and apply it with purity and sincerity. Let your femininity unfold and blossom naturally, just as a fruit tree blossoms in the springtime. If your husband should ever suspect that you are insincere or just acting a role, he will not be able to respond fully to you. Your relationship will not bear the wonderful fruit possible with fascinating womanhood. It is important to note that fascinating womanhood is an immensely powerful force for good in your marriage, although it gives the power to manipulate men. I urge you, however, to strongly resist any temptation to abuse it in this way.

In your marriage, you will certainly come to realize that you have made some mistakes. Please learn to forgive yourself, as there is nothing to be gained in continuing to blame yourself. Mistakes are learning experiences and stepping stones to future success. Real joy in life can only be experienced by first passing through sorrow. As the poet Khalil Gibran wrote: "When you are joyous, look deep into your heart and you shall find it is only that which has given you sorrow that is giving you joy....The deeper that sorrow carves into your being, the more joy you can contain."

Fascinating Womanhood: Lesson from Cathy and Dick's Conversation

One Friday evening at 8.30, Cathy ordered her children, David and Alex, off to bed and then drove around to her friend's house and borrowed a lawnmower. As she was driving back home, Dick, her husband from whom she had separated, phoned the house. Alex took the call and chatted to his father until his mother came home. Cathy arrived home a few minutes later and parked her car in the driveway. As she struggled to lift the heavy mower out of the car boot, she had great difficulty and lost her temper with it. When she finally walked into the house, she found David still lying on the floor watching TV. Cathy exploded. "David!" she yelled, "I told you to turn that thing off and go to bed! Why can't you do as you are told? Turn it off now!"

"Alex was watching too," said David sullenly, getting up to switch it off.

Cathy saw Alex sitting at the dining room table, hanging up the phone. "And who do you think you are ringing this time of the night?" she demanded.

"That was Dad," said Alex. "He has just bought himself a cell phone and was waiting to speak to you, but he heard you screaming at David and said goodbye and hung up."

Cathy was horrified. Dick had often complained about her bad temper and harsh voice. "Did he say anything else?"

"Yes. He said, 'Oh no! She hasn't changed a bit.'"

"Well, if you kids would only do as you are told, I wouldn't have to lose my temper! Your father complains about me screaming at you, and it's all your fault! Now get off to bed, both of you!"

Cathy felt utterly miserable as she prepared for bed. She wanted to phone Dick and explain, but she did not have his new cell phone number. She would have to wait until Monday and phone him at work. She felt depressed all weekend. Perhaps all her efforts so far had been undone in those few angry seconds. She shared her feelings with her friend Ami at church on Sunday. "You can't blame the children, Cathy," said Ami. ""It is your bad temper that is the problem, not them. Men don't mind if we quietly lose our temper for a good reason, but they can't stand hearing angry voices or yelling. It is just not feminine. It is too masculine. Men want us to be much better than they are. They want us to be refined, and cheerful, and gentle, and feminine." "Now, whatever you do, don't make excuses to Dick. Don't blame the children. Just apologize humbly."

On Monday morning, before leaving for school, Cathy sent Alex out to wait in the car. David had already left for school on his bike. She then phoned Dick, hoping he was already at work.

"Good morning, Jarden's Auto Services." It was Dick's voice.

"Mrs Jarden here," said Cathy brightly, trying not to sound nervous.

"Oh! Hi, Cathy," said Dick. He sounded cheerful.

"I rang to say I'm sorry, Dick, for yelling the other night when you rang. I know I've got a bad temper, and I' m going to learn to keep it under control."

"That is all right Cathy. I'm glad you are trying ... I've been reading your two letters to me, Cathy ... They make me feel ... well, sort of..."

Cathy couldn't be certain, but it sounded as if Dick were fighting back tears. His voice became emotional. "When I rang you on Friday night, I really felt my old love for you, Cathy, and I wanted to tell you. But when I heard those angry words, well ... my love just seemed to shrivel up again." Dick's voice broke. Cathy could hear him sniffing.

"He is weeping!" she thought. "Oh, Dick, I love you. I'm sorry. I really am! I promised you I would be a wonderful wife, and I will if you'll let me."

"Cathy, it has to be different if I come back. There have been too many hurts." Dick's voice sounded more composed now.

"Tell me what you want, Dick. Tell me what upsets you. I won't be offended, honestly I won't. Please tell me."

"Well, it is mostly your grouchy mouth. You really want me to be honest? Okay, I will. So many things you say hurt, Cathy. You don't seem to realize how much they hurt. And when I hear you yelling angry words, well, my love just shrivels up inside."

"What else, Dick? Please tell me."

"Well ... there is your smoking. I don't know why you have to smoke. It pongs the house. It is not a good example for David and Alex. And those black trousers you wear all the time ... I mean, when Ami came in last week, she looked great."

Cathy was hurting, but she was determined to keep going. This was the first time Dick had opened up to her since their courting days.

"I agree, Dick. Please let me know everything."

"Well, there's your hair. I love it long and shiny, and now it's short and frizzy like a man's. You know I like it long. And you have let yourself get a bit flabby. You know, fat rolls don't look very sexy."

"Is there anything else?" asked Cathy, desperately hoping there wouldn't be. "I've given up smoking and started my running again."

"No, there's nothing else that bothers me. I mean, I'm not perfect; I know that. It's just your mouth, mostly. The way you criticize everybody and shout and moan about things. I hate coming home from work when you are in one of your grouchy moods. And you could show a bit of appreciation for me now and again. I've worked hard for you and the kids over the years, and now I've got my own business. I felt good the other night when you said you liked my van. That's the first time in years I can remember you saying something nice about me. And your letters are nice, Cathy. They even brought tears to my eyes. I don't mind admitting that. Look, I've got a customer coming, I d better go," he said.

"Okay, Dick. Goodbye," she answered slowly.

Cathy walked out of the house, stunned, hurt, and somehow elated, all at once. "Knowing the problem is half the solution," she thought. Well, now she knew the problem, or rather, the problems. And her notes had made Dick cry! She hadn't known Dick to cry for years. She suddenly felt an exuberant thrill of excitement run up her spine.

What lessons can be learnt from this very emotional conversation? Certainly, it is clear that Cathy's neglect of Dick's needs is causing the failure of their marriage relationship. Millions of marriages in the world fail today because women fail to understand the man's masculinity. It may seem as though women sacrifice their femininity in doing so, but the rewards are rich. They will be rewarded many, many times over. It's like planting a seed. You can plant just one tiny apple seed and soon be rewarded with bucketfuls of apples, year after year – that is what fascinating womanhood is like. When you live up to the laws of fascinating womanhood, the love and devotion of your husband will know no bounds – he will even worship you.

Cecily Mwaniki

Serenity and Fascinating Womanhood

It is important to note that men deeply admire inner serenity and goodness in their wives. Wives must develop these traits if they want their husbands to love them deeply. Men expect their wives to be better than they are, to be more cheerful, to be kinder, more forgiving, more caring, and more spiritual. It is difficult for a man to love a sullen, resentful woman, a promiscuous one, or a noisy, argumentative one who is always yelling at the kids. But a cheerful, serene wife, one who is good and noble in her personality, is highly attractive to a man. She meets a deep need for virtue and wholesomeness in his life. He needs such a wife to create the peaceful and feminine home atmosphere so necessary to renew his spirit. He wants a woman like this to be the mother of his children, and children need a mother like this if they are to develop into warm, caring adults. It is disappointing to husbands when wives lower their standards.

But how does a woman become serene? It does not come from within, but it is the end result of goodness. Serenity and goodness go hand in hand. A woman cannot have serenity unless she has a clear conscience. She can create a serene spirit within and learn to become pure, more good-natured, and the kind of a woman that inspires and uplifts a man – a woman that he can respect, cherish, and even adore. The question to be asked, therefore, is, how does a woman regain her serenity? This question can only be answered by understanding what causes loss of serenity in the first place. The truth is, most women had serenity when they were children. That is what made them delightful to their fathers. However, they somehow lost this as they became older, mainly because we all lose our childlike humility and start listening to our consciences instead, and then we replace that by doing wrong things. The end result is that we lose respect for ourselves and are not able to control our weaknesses; we give in to anger and yell at our children and our parents as teenagers; we tell lies; we steal; we criticize; we gossip; we become jealous. All these things destroy our goodness and, of course, our serenity

When women lose their serenity, they compromise love for their husbands and the entire family. It is important to know that when a woman is serene and cheerful, her husband's love knows no bounds. Therefore, a woman must learn to safeguard her serenity by controlling her emotions before they get the better of her and steal her serenity. If her emotions are good, and her thoughts are pure, her actions should be good, as well.

An Example of the Ideal Impact of Fascinating Womanhood

When I was a kid, my mum liked to make breakfast food for dinner every now and then. And I remember one night in particular, when she had made breakfast after a long, hard day of work. On that evening so long ago, my mum placed a plate of eggs, sausages, and extremely burnt biscuits in front of my dad. I remember waiting to see if anyone noticed! Yet all my dad did was reach for a biscuit, smile at my mum, and ask me how my day had been at school. I don't remember what I told him that night, but I do remember watching him smear butter and jelly on that biscuit and eat every bite. When I got up from the table that evening, I remember hearing my mum apologize to my dad for burning the biscuits. And I will never forget what he said: "Honey, I love burnt biscuits."

Later that night, I went to kiss Daddy goodnight, and I asked him if he really liked his biscuits burnt. He wrapped me in his arms and said, "Your mummy put in a hard day at work today, and she is real tired. And besides – a little burnt biscuit never hurt anyone!"

Life is full of imperfect things and imperfect people. I am not the best at very much, and I forget birthdays and anniversaries as often as anyone else does. But what I have learned over the years is that we must accept each others' faults. Choosing to celebrate each others' differences is one of the most important keys to creating a healthy, growing, and lasting relationship.

That is what fascinating womanhood does to fascinating manhood. My prayer for you today is that you learn to take the good, the bad, and the ugly parts of your life and lay them at the feet of God. This is because, in the end, He is the only one who will give you a relationship where a burnt biscuit isn't a deal-breaker.

When all is said and done, *fascinating manhood* understands that women have energy that amazes them. Women meet difficulties and manage serious problems while remaining cheerful, loving and joyous; they smile when they want to cry out, sing when they want to shed tears, cry when they are happy, and laugh when they are nervous. They battle for what they believe in; they rebel against injustice; they do not accept no for an answer when they think there is a better solution; they deny themselves to keep the family sustained; they go to the doctor with an anxious friend; they love unconditionally. Men are amazed even more when they watch them cry when their children achieve success and rejoice at the good fortune of their friends. They are happy when they hear talk of a birth or marriage; their hearts are bruised when a friend dies; they suffer from the loss of a dear person; they are strong when they think they have no more energy; they know that a hug and a kiss can heal a wounded heart. There is no doubt that women have a fault – it is that they forget their own worth. As a woman, I challenge you today to remind your women friends to remember what wonderful creatures they are – and remind the men, too, because they sometimes need to remember this fact!

One important thing for women to remember, if they are to live in tune with fascinating womanhood, is to by all means avoid a critical spirit, even when someone has been critical to them. This will lead them to finding favour in their husbands, and above all, in God.

The Unwanted Virtuous Woman

What you are about to read may change your life! Making the choice to read further will expose you to ideas that may cause you to think and act differently.

For hundreds of years, preachers in Christian pulpits have preached the Bible's concept of a virtuous woman. They have eloquently expostulated on perhaps the most colourful description of a woman in the Bible, found in Proverbs 31:10-31. There is no other Biblical passage that makes both women and men so proud of how God values women and their role in the home and society. The virtuous woman especially stands out today in contrast to the "modern woman", the product of the feminist movement. The closing verse of the passage beautifully encapsulates the virtuous woman with these poignant words: "Many women do noble things, but you surpass them all. Charm is deceptive, and beauty is fleeting; but a woman who fears the Lord is to be praised. Give her the reward she has earned, and let her works bring her praise at the city gate". Have you ever wondered why there is no specific passage about the *virtuous man*? I submit that the virtuous woman of Proverbs 31 stands as an ideal example of God's woman today, viewed from such facets as wife, mother, member of society, manufacturer, merchant, and landowner

The writer of the "virtuous woman" (wife) passage begins with a question: "Who can find a virtuous wife?". When we compare this question with the final verse of the passage, it is clear that there were wives at the time who were not virtuous or noble. Secondly, note that the passage uses the word *wife*, because traditionally all women were required to get married. However, it will not do injustice to the passage to use the words *woman* or *wife* interchangeably. Thirdly, the word *virtuous* can be substituted with the word *noble*, indicating that the scope of the passage is not limited to the traditional sexual or "feminine" concept of a woman. Fourthly, the characteristics mentioned could be a description of a single woman. We can rightly ask the question, how could a woman do all these things? The passage seems to be a composite picture of the freedom and rights of women, how God values them, and how they should be valued by their husbands.

I am sure you have heard the saying "A woman's place is in the home". I am suggesting that a proper study of the virtuous woman in Proverbs 31 gives us the idea that a woman's role is *not* in the home. Let me conjecture that another statement to balance the picture is "A man's role includes also being in the home". Does that make us feel uncomfortable? For many years, teachers, community leaders, motivational speakers, and even ministers of the gospel have talked about what a good woman should be by quoting Proverbs 31:10-31, while they prefer their women to live the restricted lifestyle of Paul's Ephesians 5 women. Not many of us are ready for the kind of woman described in Proverbs 31.

What Is the Meaning of Virtuous Woman?

The word *virtuous*, in more modern translations, means *noble*. The word noble forces us to think about women differently. It is also used to describe force and strength of an individual. Therefore, if there is anything to strengthen mind and body, think of these things. The passage in Proverbs 31 could therefore more accurately read "Who can find a woman of strength in mind and body?" or "Who can find a woman of skill?" or "Who can find a woman of substance and capability?" These interpretations certainly place a new light on the passage. It helps us to think of a woman not as a sexual property, as the word virtuous tends to denote, but as a person of great mental and physical ability.

How Can You Describe A Noble Woman?

Noble woman, as described in Proverbs 31, has skill and strength. The husband fully leans on her and fully trusts her. Not only does she make clothing and buy food, but she also engages in real estate transactions, viniculture business, and cottage industry. Both the husband and the children of this woman praise her for her industriousness. Her earning power allows her husband to be "known in the city gates and take his seat among the elders of the land". The three outstanding roles of this noble woman are as follows:

- She speaks wisdom.
- She watches the affairs of her household.
- She considers a field and buys it.

It is unfortunate that even in the twenty-first century there are parts of the world where women are legally not allowed to do any of the above. In other places, they not allowed even to get an education.

The Paradox

What type of a woman or wife would you like to be? Would you rather be the woman/wife described with freedom, rights, and equality, or the woman/wife with no privileges, rights, or freedoms? I suggest that we love to talk about and be like the noble woman in Proverbs 31, who was a woman of strength in mind and body; we prefer to have the easy way of traditional weak, uneducated, restricted-by-law woman. However, many women have a long way to go in letting go of the concept of the traditional woman and accepting the liberated woman of Proverbs 31 who speaks wisdom and gives faithful instructions. Many men of the twenty-first century have freed women of the slavery of the past traditions and given them the right to own property, vote, get an education, state their opinions freely, and help build the community. This means the men are ready and have already accepted the "noble woman of strength, skill, and capability". I challenge *fascinating womanhood* to embrace this and with humility to build the family and the nation. This will easily lead to developing the most-needed unwanted virtuous man in the society.

I would hope that the Christian businessman or woman, whether lowest on the corporate totem pole or the chief executive officer, would be distinguished from the rest, not only by conscientious work but also by graciousness, by simple kindness, by an unassuming manliness, and above all, by a readiness to serve. We need the power that comes from being certain that God is there and being so sure of His love that we can work on in confidence at the task before us.

Some Useful Insights: Types of Wives – What Type Are You?

Party Wife

This is the woman who:

- Is very mobile and sociable
- Is always attending one function after the other (every wedding, bridal shower, kitchen top-up, office function, etc.)
- Is barely at home on weekends to have time with her husband and family
- Can spend family food money on gifts

Dictionary Wife

This is the woman who:

- Doesn't take suggestions: the way she thinks is the way she is
- Allows no changes; the way she knows is the way she maintains things
- Is very orderly and becomes angry when things are misplaced in the home set-up

Unprepared Wife

This is the woman who:

- Is very spoiled by her parents (she may be from rich parents or be the only girl in the family of many boys)

- Is lazy about doing household work
- Loves spending money shopping or on trivial girlish things
- Sees her husband as a houseboy

Office Wife

This is the woman who:

- Is so career minded that her family does not matter
- Is always using career as an excuse for not being at home for her family
- Doesn't respect her husband and makes educated women look bad
- Thinks a husband is not important, because she can support herself

Complaining Wife

This is the woman who:

- Always looks sick and downtrodden
- Loves to complain about everything (husband, children, relatives, or even the weather)
- Is always afraid and lives in anxiety

Headmistress Wife

This is the woman who:

- Puts herself in charge of the family, even when the husband is the sole provider of the home

- Treats everyone as a child, including her husband and visitors
- Is very pushy and will punish her husband for any trivial thing

Boxing Wife

This is the woman who:

- Is very offensive and sometimes can be violent
- Likes shouting and nagging
- Believes in fire for fire

Dustbin Wife

This is the woman who:

- Is very dirty and unkempt
- Is very unorganized and confused
- Is very lazy about everything except gossiping
- Leaves everything to the servants or the children

Insecurity Wife

This is the woman who:

- Is very protective of her husband
- Is very jealous and sees every woman as a threat
- Sees her husband's friends as bad company

- Doesn't let anyone discipline her child, even a teacher
- Scares her husband's family, friends, and workmates

Good Wife

This is the woman who:

- Is the virtuous wife Proverbs 31 describes
- Is caring, loving, and very smart
- Is very helpful and can even handle the husband's business in his absence
- Provides spiritual guidance to the children
- Is very understanding and full of self-esteem

You have chosen to be the kind of a wife you currently are; the good news is that you can always change/determine to be a virtuous woman.

The Unwanted Virtuous Man

Virtuous men free themselves from the clutches of tradition; however, many refuse to change. Consequently, society seems to glorify the adulterous, drug pushing, womanizing, aggressive man. The virtuous man, therefore, can be described as one:

- Who keeps his brain clean of mind-altering drugs
- Who is not afraid to cry
- Who does not cheat on his wife
- Who can say sorry to the child he hurts
- Who does not allow tradition, society, or friends to determine his way of life or the way he treats women, children, or his male friends
- Who is not concerned about what others may think of him
- Who is honest and open at all times and a man of personal integrity
- Who values and respects womanhood

Do we really want such virtuous men? Philosophically, we do. On the other hand, our traditions and language say no. The following are the reasons that tell me we do not want the virtuous men.

Men who go against the grain and do not fit into what is considered to be normal behavior by their peers are usually not promoted on the job. It does not matter if they are most productive employees or if they are always on time and respectful to their superiors. If they do not play the political games or join in the social nondeaux, they are out of the "good old boys" club, and their lives are forever limited (or so they think).

Men who have lots of children with multiple partners are considered "real men". In fact, we often find ways of excusing the indiscriminate sexual behavior of these men. A woman who goes around and flirts with men will most likely be called a bitch or whore. But a man who can sweet-talk a woman or have sex with whomever he chooses is "a cool brother".

If a single male executive gets a woman pregnant, we celebrate. We buy cigars and chocolates for the "good old boys" club. When a single female executive gets pregnant, we fire her or cry shame, shame. Virtuous men get nobody pregnant, so they cannot join the celebration. Most times they empathize with the hurting females.

Traditional fathers are free to spend all the time they want after work with the "good old boys" club. They drink beers and smoke cigars together. They play late-night dominoes. These so-called faithful fathers and husbands are free to flirt with other women. When they come home after midnight each night, they feel that their wives have no right to ask where they've been or what they've been doing. The true dad who goes straight home from work, plays with his children, and talks with his wife is considered to be a misfit. In fact, most men feel uncomfortable around him.

Certainly, these are only a few of the many ways I can think of that indicate that twenty-first-century society might not be ready for the golden era of virtuous men. But we must get ready for the new breed of noble men, because the future of our nation depends on them. Too long have we rewarded the morally starved, the mediocre, the power-crazed, the perverted, and the unfaithful man.

The good news is that there are ways of distinguishing the virtuous man from the traditional man.

Firstly, the virtuous man is spiritually astute. He is in genuine search for his creator, Jesus, the one man who was sexually pure all His life. He is externally connected by prayer to His Father and deeply engrossed in the written word of the Bible. The traditional man laughs at his fellow males who go to the altar to surrender all to Jesus, and he would not be found reading the Bible even if the lights were out. Check out our churches today. Who are mostly filling the pews?

Secondly, the virtuous man is developing himself in knowledge. He believes that reading builds a person and education is the door to the truth and life. He happily seeks ways to expand his knowledge through either formal post-secondary education or on-the-job professional development. On the other hand, the traditional man says that education is for weaklings.

I can assertively say that our nation is hurting for the need of men who can make a difference, men who are not afraid of being laughed at. On the other hand, the loud voice of traditionalism seems to be masking the pain of indifference. Since change is so painful, the chance that the members of virtuous men will increase can only depend on the strength and the stick-to-it-iveness of the few who are noble and pure.

Again I ask, do we really want the virtuous man? Would we allow him to be himself? Would we allow him to live freely outside the box of rigid traditionalism? Are we willing to change our concept of what it is to be a man? What type of man will merge successfully into the new millennium? Is it the traditional man, or is it the virtuous male? Think on these things. To add a little more heat to the discussion: men, take the Bible and read Proverbs 31:10–31, and while reading, change the gender of the passage from feminine to masculine.

Some Useful Insights: Types of Husbands – What Type Are You?

Bachelor Husband

This is the man who:

- Loves to do things on his own without consulting his wife
- Loves to hang around with his friends rather than his wife
- Is not very serious about married life

Acidic Husband

This is the man who:

- Is always angry
- Is violent
- Is moody and dominating
- Is very dangerous

Slave-Driver Husband

This is the man who:

- Feels like and wants to be treated like a king
- Treats his wife like a slave
- Loves his wife as a slave
- Loves his wife to perform old-tradition gestures of respect to him
- Doesn't like to be called by his first name

Every Woman's Husband

This is the man who:

- Is a husband to every woman
- Loves and cares for other women more than his own
- Even when not in relationships, he likes giving money to different women but not to his wife
- Has more female friends than male

Dry Husband

This is the man who:

- Is very moody
- Is very stingy
- Doesn't consider the wife's emotions
- Doesn't like putting energy into the relationship to make it enjoyable
- Doesn't have any sense of humor

'Panado' Husband

This is the man who:

- Uses his wife as a problem solver
- Loves his wife when he needs something from her, and after that she is useless to him
- Is very clever, knows his wife's weaknesses, and capitalizes on them

Parasite Husband

This is the man who:

- Is lazy and doesn't love to work; he often chooses his wife because of her money
- Is very loving but uses his wife's money and resources to cheat on her with her girlfriends
- Has no initiative and doesn't even try to help his wife with household responsibilities.

Baby Husband

This is the man who:

- Is very irresponsible and childish
- Cannot make decisions without asking his mother or other relatives
- Rushes back to his parents when something is wrong instead of discussing it with his wife
- Wants his wife to care for him as his mother did
- Always compares his wife with his mother

Visiting Husband

This is the man who:

- Is more often at work than at home
- Comes home as if he is visiting or as if his home is a lodge

- Tries hard to provide the material needs of his wife and family but has no time to give them

Good Husband

This is the man who:

- Is caring and loving
- Provides material and emotional needs for his family
- Always makes time for his family
- Guides his home spiritually
- Is very responsible and treats his wife as a partner and a helper

You have chosen to be the kind of a husband you currently are; the good news is that you can always change/ determine to be a virtuous man.

CHAPTER 3:

WOMEN AND FAMILY WELL-BEING

A woman is the full circle; within her is the power to create, nurture and transform; life shrinks or expands in proportion to one's courage. The key to change is to let go of fear

(Diane Mariechild)

Hindrances and Solutions to Women's Contribution to Family Well-Being

Women have come a long way through the years, both socially and economically, and the journey still continues, even in the twenty-first century. These changes of economic and social progress are a constant reminder for women that changes that take place on a personal level, every day, in small doses, add up to dramatic family, societal, and cultural shifts over time. This implies that women have a very important role to play for individual family well-being, which then leads to societal well-being.

In a world where women can be anything, achieve anything, and do anything, it is interesting how many still are held back by a lack of confidence. This ends up adversely affecting their families' well-being, as women are the backbone of the family and the society at large. The following are some confidence builders from some seemingly super confident women, given during interviews on how they worked on their fears and got their acts together.

- The truth is that most people are mainly concerned with themselves. Your own failures or successes, however painful or wonderful to you, are never really that high on anyone else's radar.

- Follow your own North Star. You alone know what you are good at and what feels like the right course to take for you and the family.

- That doesn't mean you have permission to stay in your comfort zone. Challenge yourself – but against your own standards, not against everyone else's.

- Brevity is the soul of everything. Short speeches are received better than long ones. A brief note makes the point faster than a long, rambling email. The joy of this is that everything becomes so much simpler and faster if you keep it short. Above all, keep your CV down to one side of A4 paper – it will have much more impact.

- Dress as if you mean business. Good grooming tells people you take yourself seriously, and other people will take their cue from that.

- And remember, even a humiliating snafu need not be a disaster. Every time I am called upon to make a speech or a presentation, I tell myself on the way up to the podium that if I should trip over and fall flat on my face, at least I will have given everyone in the audience a night to remember.

Relationship psychologist Susan Quilliam set out five ways to get confidence from those around you, namely:

1. Focus on positives. Notice – and remember – the times when people respond to you well, when they smile, take you seriously, and relax in your company.

2. Change negative thinking. Catch yourself in self put-downs, or ask those close to you to challenge you when they catch you. Then think – or even say aloud – a positive

statement, such as "I have several good friends", rather than "No one loves me".

3. Learn to say no. Politely refuse or deflect one request a day – just for practice. And make one request a day of someone else. Relationships thrive on giving as well as taking, and others will warm up to you if they feel they can give to you.

4. Resist attacks. List times, recent or past, when you were disliked, excluded, or bullied. Realize that the people who ill-treat you do so because of their own insecurity and not because of your invalidity.

5. Go for heart-lift. Identify good relationships – the ones that leave you confident rather than depleted. Schedule regular meet-ups with these people – and get a regular injection of heart-lift rather than heart-sink.

Consider this astute quote by Eleanor Roosevelt: "No one can make you feel inferior without your consent."

The key to long-term happiness and confidence is learning. Many people are not naturally confident, but learning makes them so. What counts is not how bright they are but how determined they are to expand their minds. As well-stated by Oprah Winfrey, "It is confidence in our bodies, minds and spirits that allows us to keep looking for new adventures, new directions to grow in, and new lessons to learn – which is what life is all about."

At the end of every day, take a few moments to identify three things that went well for you and contemplate your role in them. It can build self-esteem, improve your well-being, and even decrease depression, says Dr Ilona Boniwell, senior lecturer in Positive Psychology at the University of East London. By all means, say no to the quick fix. Write a list of things you like doing for yourself, and schedule them in. Do everything you can to make them happen. Research shows that taking time for yourself can substantially improve how you feel – it is much better for you than going for a quick fix, like a glass of wine.

Be altruistic. Taking time to volunteer, even for a few hours a week, will benefit you, as well as others. Volunteering has been shown to boost mental and physical health, combat depression, and help people live longer.

Be a profitable woman to your husband, your children, your parents, and above all, to your master, Jesus Christ. You need comforters in your life – people you can call who will not judge you. The challenge to you is, who are *you* comforting or uplifting? By failing to be responsible for someone, you are living as a liability, and most likely you will die as one. Avoid the feelings that you cannot comfort anybody because of something that is confronting you now. These confrontations have not come to break you but rather to build you – it is because of the potential you have to overcome it. The adversity you are facing has only come to review your potential and take you to greatness.

Imagine a new you. How? Without thinking too hard, write down a list of the way you would *like* to be. Think, "If I had more time, I would … If I had more energy, I would … If I were ten years younger, I would …". It is not about status, money or appearance, but about who you are and could be. Once you have your list, identify the first step to take towards your best self, and make it happen. It is by boosting your confidence that you victoriously carry through your family in this life. Above all else, be a praying woman, and be the kind of woman who will determine every morning to say you are too blessed to start complaining and throwing pity parties.

Women and Finances in the Twenty-First Century

As reported by Suze Orman, the writer of *Women & Money*, women today make up nearly half of the total workforce, and their income has soared dramatically by 63 per cent over the past thirty years. According to Orman's report, women bring in half or more of the income in the majority of U.S. households, with 40 per cent of companies being owned by women. However, according to a survey in 2006, commissioned by Allianz Insurance, 90 per cent of the women who participated rated themselves as feeling insecure when it came to their finances. In the same survey, nearly half the respondents said that the prospect of ending up a bag lady had crossed their minds. Then a 2006 Prudential Financial poll found that only 1 per cent of the women surveyed gave themselves an A when rating their knowledge of financial products and services. Two-thirds of women had not talked with their husbands about such things as life insurance and preparing a will. Nearly 80 per cent of women said they would depend on social security in their golden years. Did you also know that women are nearly twice as likely as men to retire in poverty? How sad! How can this be?

We see that women still don't want to take responsibility when it comes to their money – regardless of the gains in their financial status. Although they are making more money than ever before, they are not making the most of their earnings. This means, for example, that their retirement money sits in cash, because they have not figured out how to invest it properly. They have convinced themselves that they will be working forever, so the value of each paycheck becomes meaningless – after all, there will always be another one. Their closets house wardrobes of powerful and stylish women, but the dirty secret is that their credit cards are maxed out, and they don't know how they are going to pay them off. However, it is not just about saving and investing, but also about not asking for a raise at work when they know they are being undervalued. It is about the fear and loathing they feel when it is time to pay the bills every month, because they don't know exactly what they have, where it is going, or why there is no more left when all is said and done. It is also about how they berate themselves all the time for not knowing more and doing more – yet they stay resigned to this feeling of helplessness and despair as time ticks away.

I know this is all depressing, but it is useful information. Women need to think more about money matters. It is a very sensitive area, and it adversely affects their families' well-being if they do not take good care of it. Just as it is in women's nature to nurture their children, spouses, partners, pets, plants, and whatever else is in their lives, so they must learn to nurture money, as well. The truth is that they do not have a relationship with their money, and therefore it is a totally dysfunctional area. Instead, women only tend to relate to it when they are in extreme, life-changing situations in which they have no choice, for example, the birth of a child, a divorce, or death. All this causes stress to the family, which could have been avoided.

Women and Savings: The A–Z of Saving Time and Saving Money

Show me a financially healthy woman, and I will show you a happy woman. There are not many who have money to burn these days, but as we all try to cut back on spending, a grim reality emerges. Often the cheaper (and greener) way to cook or clean or organize our lives takes hours out of our already-stretched day. So how do we sort the genuine time savers from the time wasters? The Good Housekeeping Institute has come up with a unique survival guide, explained below.

A+ PERFORMANCE: Perfectionism is rarely cost effective. Sometimes it makes sense to do a job slightly less well, if it means doing it more quickly. If you have no time for every bottle and duster in the cleaning cupboard, use a damp E-cloth for a quick spruce round before guests arrive. Whenever you are using the oven, think about how you could utilize the other shelves. And instead making one lasagna, make two and freeze one.

BREAK THOSE HABITS: Get rid of worthless activities that clog up your day. Don't fritter away hours watching rubbish television; only watch, record, or use catch-up TV for the shows you really love. If you have a hoarder, time spent decluttering your home will help you cut down on housework.

CREDIT CARDS: Register all your cards with an insurer, so there is just one call if your purse is stolen, compared with hours on the phone alerting each card provider.

DON'T hire someone for a job if you can do it yourself or can combine it with an activity you enjoy. Do the ironing while watching East Enders, for example, or tidy up while chatting on the phone.

ESTIMATE: work out how long it will take you to do a task. Writing a to- do list when you are snowed under will help you stay in control. Will it take five minutes, or will it take an hour? Set your deadline and stick to it.

FREE TIME: Once you have shed the tasks you hate, or that make more sense to farm out, don't waste the time you have freed up. Otherwise, everything else will expand to fill that time hole. Rather, enroll in that psychology or computer class, book those tickets, or enjoy a long bath.

GADGETS: Having the right equipment makes a job easier and quicker. A handy cleaning kit will tackle stains; sharp knives make cooking easier; and a dishwasher is more efficient and uses less water than you do.

HIRE SOMEONE ELSE: If you really hate cleaning the oven, pay an oven-cleaning service. Don't feel guilty about delegating jobs in areas where you know you fall short. If it is really not your forte, farm it out, and give someone else the chance to excel.

IRONS, WASHING MACHINES: If you are looking for new appliances, check out the Good Housekeeping Institute website: www.allaboutyou/Good-HouseKeeping-Tried-Tested/channel for best buys you can trust.

JUST IN CASE: Write down a list of important phone numbers – the doctor, babysitter, school, child minder, and plumber – and pin it to the kitchen notice board, so the information is easy to find. Get details of recommended tradesmen before you need them.

KEEP FIT: Incorporate exercise into your daily routine rather than trying to take time out to go to the gym. Walking to the shops, doing the housework, and gardening vigorously will save money, burn calories, and make you feel great.

LOCAL: Support your corner shop whenever you can, rather than driving out to – and battling – the supermarket.

MAKE A LIST: Write down items to buy during your next shopping trip as soon as you think of them, and take the list with you when you shop. You will avoid impulse buys and stop forgetting essentials.

NET WORTH – YOURS: The average wage in the United Kingdom, says the 2009 *Annual Survey of Hours and Earnings* (*ASHE*), is £20,801, with the top 25 per cent earning an average gross salary of £31,759. Whether you are salaried or not, we reckon Good Housekeeping readers' time is worth at least £16 an hour – roughly £11 net of tax. Never undervalue yourself.

ONLINE SHOPPING: This saves stacks of time, and money, too, as you won't be prone to impulse buys. Online grocery shopping costs £6 to deliver (less at peak times) plus half an hour of your time ordering and unpacking. Compare that with driving to the supermarket, slogging round the aisles for two hours, and unpacking it all when you get home. Yes, it takes a maddeningly long time to register – but it will be worth it.

PAPERWORK AND PLANNING: Organize files into a system, update your phone book, and photocopy important documents. While you may feel "I wish I had never started this", in the long run, it does save time. Chaos is a ferocious time thief. Organizing saves you the anxiety of trying to remember to do things.

QUEUEING: As a nation, we may be brilliant at it – but why queue when you don't have to? Pay for petrol up front at the pump, use self-scanning checkouts and book tickets for tourist attractions and train journeys online. It could save money, too – a ticket to Alton Towers resort for a family of four costs 20 per cent less if you buy it online.

ROUTE PLANNING: Avoid getting lost by checking your route before you set off. You will save petrol and angst, too. Print out maps from www.theaa.com/travel or www. rac.co.uk/plan-a-trip, or use an up-to-date SatNav (a global-positioning device).

SET LIMITS: Music lessons, drama, tennis, karate, spin classes, sleepovers, book clubs, coffee mornings, committees – decide what is important to you and your family, and then get rid of the rest. Be selective.

TEAMWORK: Say yes to offers of help from friends and family, if it means you can blitz the garden or redecorate a room over a weekend rather than letting it drag on or having to pay for professional help.

UNWANTED DISTRACTIONS: Don't be diverted from the day's tasks – we are talking about answering calls from salesmen, a third cup of tea, reading junk emails, or tracking bargains on eBay.

VOUCHERS: Cut out coupons from magazines or download them – the Internet is awash with discount vouchers. Try www.myvouchercodes.co.uk and www.moneysavingexpert.com.

WHY: Why spend hours comparing prices, when someone else has done it? Try sites such as www.pricerunner.co.uk, www.kelkoo.co.uk, and www.pricegrabber.co.uk for electronics; www.uswitch.com and www.moneysupermarket.com for utilities, insurance, and telecoms; and www.travelsupermarket.com and www.skyscanner.net for cheap flights.

XFACTOR: We all have our strengths. By knowing which tasks you are good at, you can achieve much more. Perhaps your partner is a whiz at math's homework and Sunday roasts, while you are better with computers and paying bills. "Vive la difference!" we say.

YOUTH OF TODAY: A recent survey by the Halifax bank showed that children get around £300 a year in pocket money – some a lot more. So don't ever feel bad about asking them to do things to help around the house.

ZZZZZ: Use all that freed-up time to relax – you will hopefully be less stressed, because you will have saved money

Why Women Cry: The Need to Boost Confidence

"Why do women cry?" a small boy asked God. This is the answer that God gave:

"When I created woman, she needed to be special. I created her shoulders strong enough to bear the weight of the world and soft enough to be comfortable. I gave her the strength to give life. I made her the kind who accepts the rejection that often comes from children, men, friends, and even other women. I gave her strength, to allow her go on when everyone else gives up. I made her the kind that takes care of her family, despite illness and fatigue. I gave her the sensitivity to love her children unconditionally, even when they have hurt her deeply. I gave her the strength to endure her husband's faults and to stay at his side without weakening. And finally, I gave her tears to shed whenever she needs them to be shed. You see, my son, the beauty of a woman is not in the clothes she wears, nor is it in her face, or in the way she does her hair. The beauty of a woman resides in her eyes. They are the door to her heart, the door behind which she resides, and it is often through her tears that you see her heart go by and lift the spirit of other people. Therefore, men, don't always wonder when you see women shed tears."

Women's Beautiful Attitude

How blessed is the woman who knows her need of God, for only then can others find a bit of heaven in her presence. Blessed is the woman who finds in sorrow the comfort of living God, who learns that although life is burdened with unhappiness, a heart overflowing with gratitude can seek and find such fullness of joy that all bitterness is crowded out. Happy is the family of the woman who possesses a gentle spirit. Her husband will place his world at her feet; her children will come often to her door. She truly listens and surely hears.

How blessed is the woman who yearns for justice and does something about it – she shares her home with the homeless, her food with the hungry, her joy with the desolate – yet she cares for the needs of her own family, including them in the sharing.

Happy is the woman who knows how to forgive, who cannot hold a grudge, and who asks others for forgiveness. Divine forgiveness shall be hers. Happy is the woman whose heart is pure, swept clean of self-pity, nagging, and complaints. In her heart is abundant love for her husband. So happy will her marriage be that others will see God in her home. Even their children shall behold Him.

How blessed is the woman who is a peacemaker, sharing neither gossip nor fault-finding. She studies her children to learn how to bring peace to them. She has self-esteem, because God is her Father. Her children respect her, because she is fair and just. She teaches them how to become members of God's family. Heavenly peace shall dwell deep within her soul.

How blessed is the woman who, waits with Christ, finds joy in waiting with her sisters in Christ. She will form bonds that will last through eternity. Can this woman be happy when she has been misunderstood, mistreated, unappreciated? Yes, for she has exchanged her will for God's peace, joy, and love, and she will be given God's crowning gift – heaven.

It is a fact that our attitudes define our lives. Life is best for those who want to live it well. Life is difficult for those who want to analyse it, and is worst for those who want to criticize it. Laugh so hard that even sorrow smiles at you. Live life so well that even death loves to see you alive. Fight so hard that even fate accepts defeat.

As a woman of substance, learn to grateful for what you have and who you are. It is gratitude that determines your altitude in life – but not your aptitude. Keep a gratitude journal, because life is full of pursuits. Stop and learn to be grateful. Thank God for your enemies, because they make you move. Remember that gratitude is an attitude that determines your altitude in life.

Cecily Mwaniki

The Balance Sheet of a Fascinating Woman's Life

Her birth is her opening balance.

Her death is her closing balance.

Her prejudiced views are her liabilities.

Her creative ideas are her assets.

Heart is her current asset.

Soul is her fixed asset.

Brain is her fixed deposit.

Thinking is her current account.

Achievements are her capital.

Character and morals are her stock in trade.

Friends are her general reserves.

Values and behavior are her goodwill.

Patience is her interest.

Love is her dividend.

Children are her bonus issues.

Education is her brand or patent.

Knowledge is her investment.

Experience is her premium account.

The aim is to tally the balance sheet accurately.

The goal is to get the best-presented-accounts award.

Fascinating Women's Marketplace for Character, Actions, and Emotions

The most destructive habit: **Worry**

The greatest joy: **Giving**

The greatest loss: **Loss of self-respect**

The most satisfying work: **Helping others**

The ugliest personality trait: **Selfishness**

The most endangered species: **Dedicated leaders**

The greatest natural resource: **Youth**

The greatest "shot in the arm": **Encouragement**

The greatest problem to overcome: **Fear**

The most effective sleeping pill: **Peace of mind**

The most crippling failure- disease: **Excuses**

The most powerful force in life: **Love**

The most dangerous act: **Gossip**

The world's most incredible computer: **The brain**

The worst thing to be without: **Hope**

The deadliest weapon: **The tongue**

The two most power-filled words: **"I can"**

The greatest asset: **Faith**

The most worthless emotion: **Self-pity**

The most beautiful attire: **A smile**

The most prized possession: **Integrity**

The most powerful channel of communication: **Prayer**

The most contagious spirit: **Enthusiasm**

The Seven Unbeatable Secrets of Happy Wives/Women

We all have sweet memories of our meticulously planned and choreographed weddings – they were perfect. But many marriages? Oops, there was no script, and somehow, many believed the honeymoon bliss would carry over into day-to-day life. But there are some really happy wives, and the following is what they have to say about the secrets of their happiness.

Remember your third partner. God has promised to stand by the two of you – forever. Stay connected to Him through prayer for and with your husband. My friend Nancy points out that prayer is a great way to resolve conflicts. She says, "When Dave and I can't agree on something, we always say, 'let's pray about it'. Praying together brings us into a common mind, where we are willing to accept God's will and more ready to compromise." Remember, God invented marriage. If you let Him, He is dedicated to creating happiness between you and your husband.

Speak up, shut up, and listen up. In other words, communicate. If your interaction with your husband never extends past "Honey, where is the remote?", there is trouble. Listening without interrupting or passing judgment on what he is saying is most important. Resist the temptation to assume that he knows what you are feeling. Remember, men are from Mars!

Judy kept her feelings inside, insisting to her girlfriends that Jack "should know how much it upsets me to have his brother over four nights a week", or she would say,

"Why should I have to tell him when I am hurt? The look on my face should be hint enough." And after years of emotional pressure building, like a shaken-up soda bottle, Judy exploded. Her marriage now lies in soggy pieces.

Lesson for Judy: deal with the problems – communicate – before you are past the point of no return. Begin by simply making an effort. Educate yourself. An incredible number of good books exist on how to communicate. All you need is a free library card. When you put new habits in place, your man will likely jump into the game with you.

Accept his quirks. Joan's husband eats loudly, and it can drive her nuts. "If he is eating, but I am not, I just have to find ways to make noise and keep busy!" And then there is Sarah, who has wiped up Phil's crumbs and set his empty juice glass in the sink every morning for thirty years. Does it still bug her? Well, sometimes. "But after complaining to some trusted girlfriends and being told their husbands are incurable too, it made it easier to chill." The bottom line is, you are not going to change everything about him that you would like to, no matter how much you try. So give it up. Remember, you have got better stuff to worry about than whether he unwinds his tube socks before they hit the laundry chute. It is important to note that you have habits that irritate him, too.

Dwell on the positive. First of all, decide to love him. Make the conscious decision to work with your marriage, grow with it, and stick with it. Your mind believes what you constantly tell it, so stop giving it negative input. Focus on your husband's good traits. Look for the little things that show he cares. You say they are not there? I bet they are. Do you take for granted that he keeps your car clean or drops you off by the mall door? Appreciate it, and tell him so. It's important to take notice of even the smallest sweet thing he does. Then learn to smooth over the really picky issues. I learned this lesson s-l-o-w-l-y during the first few weeks that James started teaching me how to drive. Ask yourself if this thing that seems so important to you will really matter twenty years from now. If the current issue will cause deep or recurring pain, get it out in the open, and work through it. If it's not going to change – and use your good sense here – get over it, and move on with your life.

Let your hair down. How long have you had the same hair style? We all thrive on continuity, but a surprise now and then spices things up. Ask him out on a date. Have a candlelight dinner and romantic music ready when he gets home from work, or slip into the shower with him. Invest in a book on creative romance, and try at least one idea each week.

Depend on yourself for your happiness. You can't expect that your husband will ever meet all of your needs. "Two becoming one" is the goal of a God-blessed union, but you are still an individual. You have an identity apart from him. Don't base your happiness on his actions. If you wait to be content until he starts being more helpful around the house, you may have a long wait. Happiness flows from your state of mind, and you have control over that. So what can you do? Make a decision to do things that give you satisfaction. For example, start gardening – inside or outside. Plan a girls' night out. Take up piano lessons. Do something for yourself.

Admire this incredible man you married. He needs to be adored, just as you do. It's like this: Your man's ego is a garden the size of Yankee Stadium, and your job is to water the flowers. So kick the gigantic sprinkler system into high gear. How? First of all, just listen to him (hang on every word, if need be). Believe it or not, you *can* care about the details of how he has engineered the new basement drain. Why? Because it's important to him, and he is important to you. Remember to brag about him to other people. Let others know how much you admire him, and he will repay you in ways you have not even thought of. And while all men possess bewildering traits that make us crazy, never put down your husband within 100 yards of other ears. As one woman put it, "If I dis him, it makes me look an idiot for marrying him. But if I praise him, it affirms my great taste." So you get to build him up – and yourself at the same time! Talk about a win-win situation.

These seven unbeatable secrets can become reality to you. Just watch – you will become a happy wife when you start practicing them. This will lead you to having a happy husband, too.

Why Women Need the Friendship of Other Women

"We women all need at least one close friend to confide in. Someone we can talk to heart to heart. Our husbands are our friends, but they can't meet all our special needs."

Most men don't like to talk too much, anyway. Research has shown that our female brains are more highly developed in verbal areas. We women can speak about 50,000 words a day before we become tired of talking. But most men can only manage about 25,000. That is one of the reasons most men don't feel like talking much when they come home after work. They have used up their quota during the day. Also, women and men have different interests. For example, how many of us women are really interested in the mechanical details of cars or the play skills of rugby players?

We realize that women in the native villages are always mingling together, washing clothes in the river and collecting water from the well. These women always look very happy on TV, just following the traditions of their mothers – they have no stress. They rarely suffer from stress. It is therefore necessary to seek the companion and the comfort of other women

Surprises of a Woman on Becoming a Mother

Mothers draw their joy from their children. It is no wonder that before a woman becomes a mother, she has all sorts of imaginings of what a wonderful, proud mother she will be. The following was the confession of one woman who for a long time had longed to be a mother but was caught by surprise when she became one:

"Before I was a mom, I never tripped over toys or forgot words to a lullaby. I didn't worry whether or not my plants were poisonous. I never thought about immunizations. I had never been puked on, pooped on, chewed on, and certainly never peed on. I had complete control of my mind and my thoughts. I slept all night. Before I was a mom, I had never held down a screaming child so doctors could do tests or give shots, never looked into teary eyes and cried, never got gloriously happy over a simple grin, or even sat up late hours at night watching a baby sleep. Before then, I had never held a sleeping baby just because I didn't want to put her down, never felt my heart break into a million pieces when I could not stop the hurt, and never known that something so small could affect my life so much. I never knew that I could love someone so much, and most of all, I never knew I would love being a mom.

"I never knew the feelings of having my heart outside my body. I didn't know that something so small could make me feel so important and happy. I had never gotten up in the middle of the night every ten minutes to make sure all was okay. Worse still, I had never known the warmth, the joy, the heartache, the wonderment, or the satisfaction of being a mom – I didn't know I was capable of feeling so much". How wonderful would it be, however, to be overwhelmed by the Grace of God, rather than by the cares of life.

Indeed, being a mother is challenging, yet rewarding. It requires wisdom, skills, and most of all, love. It is a beautiful role for a woman, on top of being a homemaker.

It is no wonder that a mother is God's love in action. She looks with her heart and feels with her eyes. A mother is the bank where her children deposit all their worries and hurts. She is also the cement that keeps her family together, and her love lasts a lifetime. There is no doubt that motherhood is the toughest twenty-four-hour, lifetime job. There is no pay, no day off, no qualifications, and no training given. It is most often unappreciated, and resignation is impossible. No wonder mothers are celebrated as terrific *Mum*s by their children!

Did You Know? (Henry David Thoreau)

Did you know that those who appear to be very strong in heart are real weak and most susceptible?

Did you know that those who spend their time protecting others are the ones that really need someone to protect them?

Did you know that the three most difficult things to say are "I love you," "I'm sorry," and "Help me"?

Did you know that those who dress in red are more confident in themselves?

Did you know that those who dress in yellow are those that enjoy their beauty?

Did you know that those who dress in black are those who want to be unnoticed and need your help and understanding?

Did you know that when you help someone, the help is returned twofold?

Did you know that it is easier to say what you feel in writing than saying it to someone in the face? But did you also know that it has more value when you say it on the face?

Did you know that when you ask for something in faith, your wishes are granted?

Did you know that you can make your dreams come true, like falling in love, staying healthy, if you ask for it by faith, and if you really knew you'd be surprised by what you could do?

Note that the language of friendship is not in words but meanings. You can, therefore, confidently say to your true friend that he gave you a whole meaning to your life. It is also important to note that if a thousand people say something is not foolish when it clearly is, it's still foolish. Trust is never dependent upon consensus of opinion.

CHAPTER 4:

HEALTH, WEALTH, AND HAPPINESS

It is health that is real wealth and not pieces of gold and silver. The first wealth is health, for he who has health has hope, and he who has hope has everything. However, many people spend their health gaining wealth and then spend their wealth regaining their health.

(Mahatma Gandhi)

What is Health, and What Does It Mean to You?

As defined by the World Health Organization (WHO), health is not merely the absence of disease or infirmity but also a state of complete physical, mental, and social well-being. This definition was further described in the World Health Organization 1986 Ottawa Charter for Health Promotion as a resource for everyday life and not just the objective of living. In simple terms, health is achieved through a combination of physical, mental, and social well-being, which together is commonly referred to as the *health triangle*. The triangle has to be complete for you to be healthy. However, as life is a problem-solving process, the triangle is not always complete. To achieve a complete triangle, it is important to be aware of the fact that life is a problem-solving process and therefore to face the problems and deal with them as they come. Take time and read the following to empower you to achieve total well-being without any monetary cost implications.

Stress: A Health Scare that Can Be Avoided

Most people experience less leisure and more daily stress, as they juggle work and career, family, and friends. In spite of life's demands, there are simple, effective, daily ways to deal with pressure. Here are sixteen ways to reduce stress during the workday.

Begin the day with a brief prayer and meditation. Rather than jumping out of bed and rushing to start your day, take between five and twenty minutes to play, meditate, read a short inspiring passage, think peaceful thoughts, or appreciate God's gift of a new, fresh day. Beginning this way gives you a sense of peace that will manifest itself all day.

Apply the wisdom of Paul to your daily living. "Whatever is noble ... whatever is pure, whatever is lovely, whatever is admirable ... think about such things" (Philippians 4: 8). Those words are a reminder to think positively. During the day, whenever you face a crisis, think *challenge*; when you face an obstacle, think *opportunity*. When you approach any stressful event with positive thoughts, this will boost your energy.

Remember, you get to make mistakes. "Many people start sinking into despair or scolding themselves unmercifully after making a mistake," observes Charlotte Davis Kasl, Ph.D., a psychologist and author of *Finding Joy*. "The important thing to remember is that anyone makes mistakes ... so ease up on yourself."

Create peaceful images in your mind. Several times during your workday, pause briefly to create a peaceful image in your mind. For example, picture yourself gently canoeing on calm, still lake, with the sun shining brilliantly. Or imagine yourself sitting quietly on a hillside, where you are completely surrounded by beautiful wildflowers.

Practice hospitality. Maintain an open-door policy in your heart for everyone you will encounter during the day. Greet everyone with a smile. This will make others feel good about being with you.

Observe your breathing. When we are relaxed, our breathing is slow and even. However, when we are anxious or upset, we tend to breathe irregularly. Pay attention to your breathing. As soon as you notice yourself becoming stressed, say to yourself "Stop." As you breathe out, smile. As you do this, let your shoulders drop, and relax your hands. Repeat this technique several times.

Take a brisk walk. Experts note that exercise is effective in burning off the excess adrenaline that fuels feelings of anxiety and stress. Exercise also releases endorphins – the body's natural chemicals that block anxiety and pain. So take a brisk walk over lunch hour. During office hours, even a brisk walk down the hallway or up a flight of stairs can help.

Change your lunch environment. Get out of the office and enjoy your noon meal in a park. Use this time to be with nature. At least once or twice a week, eat by yourself in silence. Eat slowly. Be thankful for your meal. Enjoy yourself.

Be aware of what you drink. The caffeinated drinks you drink throughout the day can be a mental health nightmare. Too much caffeine can cause shaky hands, restlessness, and irritability – all of which increase stressful feelings. Try eliminating it from your routine.

Concentrate on the task at hand, not the outcome. This is another way of learning to be less than perfect. If you find yourself fretting about a project, speak gently to yourself, saying "Here I go again worrying about the future. I'll just give this my best now." Then do that. Remember to leave the future in God's hands.

Just say no. You don't have to accept any project, every invitation to become involved, and every opportunity to attend a meeting. Accept what you need to do and what you want to do, but say "No, thank you" to other requests for your time.

Make a peace pact with yourself. As soon as you begin to feel angry, hostile, cynical, skeptical, irritable, or impatient, repeat a word that can offset the negative energy. Some examples include *peace, love, hope, joy,* and *patience.*

Relive a happy memory. The right music can take you from a highly tense state to a relaxed state in a very short time. The right music is generally instrumental rather than vocal. Many people find the sounds of nature combined with musical harmonies to be very relaxing.

Don't bring work problems home. Leave cares behind at the office. You will feel better, and you will return to work refreshed, energetic, and more creative. Saki F. Santorelli,

Ed.D., assistant professor of medicine at the University of Massachusetts Medical Centre, offers these tips: At the end of the workday, sit quietly, and consciously make the transition from work to home. When you pull into the driveway or park on the street, take a minute to orient yourself to entering your home and being with your family members. Try changing out of your work clothes when you get home. This simple act might help you to make a smoother transition into your next 'role'.

How Well Do You Cope?

Life is a problem-solving process, and the absence of problems doesn't automatically make life beautiful. It is actually healthy to experience problems, because it is when tackling them that we exercise or test our brains' health. How do *you* cope with problems or crises? Do you bounce back unscathed, or do you wither in the face of adversity? The manner in which you react to a stressful situation greatly depends on your way of coping. What do you do when the going gets tough?

Many of our coping mechanisms, such as problem solving, are consciously selected, while others, known as defense mechanisms, are largely unconscious. We use them when we are faced with a stressful situation or crisis and have to find a way to overcome it or adjust to it. Some coping strategies are adaptive (such as changing our perception), whereas others are maladaptive (such as self-medicating with alcohol and/or drugs).

Coping mechanisms. Researchers distinguish three types of coping strategies: efforts to change the situation, efforts to change your perception about the situation, and efforts to change the unpleasant emotions you experience as a result of the stress. Trying to change the *situation* usually involves problem solving: you try to remove the stressor, come up with ways to resolve the issue, or ask for advice or help from others. People who have well-developed problem-solving abilities – they can see problems as challenges and confront them directly – tend to experience less stress and fewer psychological symptoms than those who don't. Changing your *perception* (also called reframing) is another way to cope with a stressful situation to make it less threatening. For example, instead of being nervous about giving a speech, you could look at it as a conversation with a bunch of people who are interested in what you have to say. Another way to cope is to try to make yourself feel different *emotions*; you might laugh when you are nervous. Other ways include listening to music, meditating, exercising, or anything else that relieves stress or puts you in a good mood. People may also use avoidance or distraction to escape their emotional distress. Of course, as I have mentioned before, they may also engage in maladaptive behavior, such as excessive drinking or drug use. And while this may provide temporary relief, it is bound to come back and bite them in the butt later on.

Defence mechanisms. Most of the coping mechanisms I have described above are conscious or can readily be made conscious, if we call attention to them. Defence mechanisms, on the other hand, are unconscious and involve a bit of self-deception. They were first described by psychodynamic psychologists (you have heard of Freud?) as unconscious mental processes that are aimed at protecting a person from experiencing unpleasant emotions or reinforcing positive emotions. Some of the defence mechanisms often used are as follows:

- **Repression**: when unconscious mechanism keeps thoughts and memories that are too threatening from your conscious awareness

- **Denial**: when you refuse to acknowledge external realities (such as having cancer) or emotions (such as anxiety)

- **Projection**: when you attribute your own unacknowledged or unwanted feelings and thoughts onto others (for example, when you think everyone is out to deceive you, *you* may be the one with questionable ethics)

- **Reaction formation**: when you turn unacceptable feelings or impulses into their opposite (A good example is televangelist Jimmy Swaggart who, while preaching the evils of sex to millions, was regularly seeing a prostitute. His conscious repulsion toward sexuality, particularly illicit sex, apparently masked a tremendous need for it.)

- **Sublimation**: when you channel sexual or aggressive impulses into socially acceptable activities (such as changing competitiveness with your brother into competitiveness on the sports field or striving for success in your job)

- **Rationalization**: when you explain away actions in a seemingly logical way to avoid unpleasant feelings like guilt or shame

- **Passive aggression**: when you indirectly express your anger towards others (such as withholding important information from a colleague because he was promoted before you)

We use these defence mechanisms flexibly and creatively, as need arises. Mostly, using these defences is not abnormal or unhealthy. In fact, a little distortion (such as seeing yourself more positively than is warranted by reality) and denial (such as persevering despite repeated rejection and then finally succeeding) can go a long way. It is only when these defence mechanisms inhibit normal functioning that they become a problem.

If you feel that you just can't cope when the going gets tough, try to find ways of reducing your stress and enhancing your mood. For some ideas on how to bounce back and manage stress, consider consulting a psychologist who is trained to help you learn how to cope.

Why Things Look Grey When You Feel Blue

We usually describe depression as dark or sombre, and now researchers have found a possible explanation for that. Scientists at the University of Freiburg in Germany, who previously showed that depressed people have difficulty detecting black-and-white contrast differences, recently studied the link between depression and vision. The researchers measured the retinal responses to different black-and-white contrast situations in groups of depressed and non-depressed individuals. They found that depressed volunteers had significantly lower retinal nerve activity than non-depressed volunteers, diminishing their ability to perceive contrast. It made no difference whether the depressed participants were taking antidepressant medication or not. There was also a strong correlation between severity of depression and ability to detect contrast. Participants with most severe symptoms of depression had the lowest retinal responses.

According to one of the researchers, Dr Ludger Tebartz van Elst, this method could have far-reaching implications for research and clinical diagnosis of therapy for depression.

Dr John Krystal, editor of the journal *Biological Psychiatry*, where these findings were published, was quoted as saying "These data highlight the profound ways that depression alters one's experience of the world." The poet William Cowper said that "Variety's the very spice of life", yet when people are depressed, they are less able to perceive contrasts in the visual world. This loss would seem to make the world a less pleasurable place.

While these findings need to be replicated, and a casual relationship has not been established, the study reinforces the notion that depression isn't only an emotional experience. If you think that you may be depressed; if you experience changes in mood, appetite or sleep, or are no longer interested in activities you previously enjoyed, speak to a health professional.

Note that when struggling with clinical depression, many people feel the only solution is medication. However, research has found that *talk therapy* can sometimes be just as effective as medication. Talk therapy with a trained professional tends to bring more lasting recovery and fewer relapses than medication. It helps people address the interpersonal problems contributing to their sadness, and it does not have the side effects of medication.

Your Relationships and Your Health

Feeling insecure in your relationship or having trouble getting close to others may have important implications for your life, a recent study found. According to the study, by the American Psychological Association (APA), researchers from Arcadia University in Canada analysed data on 5,645 people who took part in the nationally represented survey of adults aged 18 to 60. Participants were asked to rate their relationships according to three attachment styles: secure attachment (being comfortable when close to others and depending on them); avoidant attachments (feeling uncomfortable being close to others and having difficulty trusting others); or anxious attachments (feeling needy, worrying about rejection, and finding others to be reluctant to get close to you). They were also asked about their medical histories, focusing on issues such as arthritis, chronic back and neck problems, frequent or severe headaches, other forms of chronic pain, seasonal allergies, stroke, and heart attack. In addition, participants were asked to disclose diagnoses of heart disease, high blood pressure, asthma, chronic lung disease, diabetes or high blood sugar, ulcers, epilepsy, seizures, or cancer, as well as psychological disorders. After controlling for other variables that could account for the health conditions mainly defined by pain (such as frequent or severe headaches), they found that those with anxious attachment styles were at higher risk for several health conditions, including stroke, heart attack, high blood pressure, chronic pain, and ulcers.

According to the lead author, Lachlan A. McWilliams, Ph.D., these findings suggest that insecure attachment may be a risk factor for a wide range of health problems, particularly cardiovascular diseases. Longitudinal research on this topic is needed to determine whether insecure attachment predicts the development of cardiovascular disease and the occurrence of cardiovascular events such as heart attacks. As McWilliams further says, the findings also raise the possibility that interventions aimed at improving attachment security could also have positive health outcomes.

If you have trouble getting close to other people and trusting them – if you feel uncomfortable around them or worry about rejection quite often – it may be a good idea to speak to a counselor or a psychologist about how to relate to others. A healthy attachment style may not only have positive health outcomes, as this study suggests, but it will also boost your resilience and improve your quality of life.

Kindness and Its Health Benefits

In brief, it seems that there is something in it for you if you help someone else. Kindness holds mental and physical health benefits. And it doesn't take enormous efforts on your part, either. Just try, and see how much you can benefit by lending a hand.

In our what-is-in-it-for-me society, kindness is a rarity. As most of us view the costs (in terms of time, effort, and so on) of helping someone else as outweighing the benefits, we simply don't bother. But research suggests that altruism may not be completely selfless, after all. In fact, the helper may benefit more than the person being helped.

Studies show that helping others contributes to the maintenance of good health, and it can diminish the effects of diseases and disorders. According to the Random Acts of Kindness Foundation, some of the following benefits may be experienced.

- A rush of euphoria, followed by a longer period of calm, may occur after we perform a kind act. This is often referred to as a "helper's high" and involves physical sensations and the release of the body's natural painkillers, the endorphins. This initial rush is then followed by a longer-lasting period of improved emotional well-being.

- Stress-related health problems improve after we perform kind acts. Helping reverses feelings of depression, supplies social contact, and decreases feelings of hostility and isolation that can cause stress, overeating, ulcers, etc. A drop in stress may, for some people, decrease the constriction within the bronchi of the lungs that leads to asthma attacks.

- Helping can enhance our feelings of joyfulness, emotional resilience, and vigour and can reduce the unhealthy sense of isolation.

- A decrease in both the intensity and the awareness of physical pain can occur.

- The incidence of attitudes, such as chronic hostility, that negatively arouse and damage the body is reduced.

- The health benefits and sense of well-being return for hours or even days whenever the helping act is remembered.

- An increased sense of self-worth, greater happiness, and optimism, as well as a decrease in feelings of helplessness and depression, is achieved.

- Once we establish an *affiliative connection* with someone – a relationship of friendship, love, or some sort of positive bonding – we feel emotions that can strengthen the immune system.

- Regular club attendance, volunteering, entertaining, or faith group attendance is the happiness equivalent of getting a degree or more than doubling your income.

We can therefore deduce that

- adopting an altruistic lifestyle is a critical component of mental health.
- the practice of caring for strangers translates to immense immune and healing benefits.

It is not necessary to carry out monumental acts of kindness to experience these benefits, either. In fact, it has been found that brief, small, regular acts of kindness lead to the highest levels of well-being. It has also been found that such small, pleasurable experiences can more than offset any negative health effects brought about by life's stressful events, regardless of their magnitude.

But what exactly are "brief, small, regular acts of kindness", and how do you incorporate them into your already-crammed schedule?

It is not difficult to incorporate kindness into your everyday life. You don't even really have to put time aside to do so. Simply do it while you are doing something bigger. But for now, here are a few ideas that you can start doing today, if you are not already doing them:

Smile and say hello to someone you don't know. This could be someone at work, at the grocery store, or another traffic-frustrated commuter.

Let someone jump the queue. If you are standing in line at the bank, the canteen, or the shop, and you notice someone who seems to be in a hurry, why not let him jump the queue?

Treat a stranger. Leave enough money in the vending machine for the next person to get a free treat.

Share the load. Help someone who is struggling to carry heavy bags or a big load.

Treat someone to fresh fruit. It is healthy, it is delicious, and it might just make someone's day.

Write a thank-you note to someone who has influenced your life positively. Everyone appreciates the knowledge that they have made an impact on someone else.

Hand out kindness coupons. Give friends and family kindness coupons they can redeem for a special favor.

Drop off a plant or cookies at your local police station. These men and women are often only confronted with the negative aspects of life. Show them that you appreciate their contribution to your community.

Organize a clothing drive at work. Most people have items they want to discard, but often they don't have the time or don't know where it is needed. Ask them to bring it to work and then drop it off at a shelter or charity organization.

These are just a few ideas to get you going. Try it, or any other thought of generosity, for one week – and notice what happens as a consequence. Chances are you will notice that kindness has a way of catching on.

Married Mothers on the Best Wicket

In brief, some say we cannot have it all, but recent research says that women who are married, have children, and are employed are less likely to suffer from poor mental health. It seems that being well-integrated promotes good mental health.

Marry, have children, get a job, and be a woman. If you can manage all four, you would make it into the demographic group most likely to be free of mental disorder, according to a recent study on the distribution of such conditions.

A study reported in *Age*, a journal that publishes research on aging, suggests that women who are married, have children, and are in the workforce are the least likely to suffer mental disorders, while unmarried, childless, unemployed men are the most at risk.

David de Vaus, associate professor in sociology at La Trobe University and senior research adviser at the Australian Institute of Family Studies, said the research showed that marriage, or having a partner, acted as a "protective device" to some extent, because it meant greater support. He said marriage has in the past been cast as an exacerbating factor in the development of mental disorders, especially in light of the rising divorce rate. This has led to some neglect of the positives that flow from being married.

The analysis is based on recently released figures from the Australian Bureau of Statistics' national survey, *Mental Health and Wellbeing of Adults*, in which more than 10,000 people were interviewed. It is the first comprehensive study of the link between relationships and mental health since the 1960s. Research suggested that marriage improved men's mental health – but not that of their wives. However, Professor de Vaus said the data that was collected then had enormous gaps in it, and so you really could not conclude one way or the other.

The new report shows that married people are less likely to suffer mental disorders, that divorced or separated people are the most prone to mood and anxiety disorders, and that never-married adults are most susceptible to drug and alcohol abuse. Regardless of mental status, women are almost twice as likely to suffer anxiety disorders and men are twice as likely to suffer substance abuse. People who already had mental-health problems found it harder to get partners in the first place – or to stay partnered – but having a partner or having children tended to stabilize people.

In conclusion, Professor de Vaus was quoted as saying "The more anchors both men and women have, the better integrated they are; the better their mental health."

Raising Healthy Kids

As parents struggle to balance busy work schedules, their children are often being shaped by a number of less-than-ideal influences. Children are constantly exposed to advertising, media, and peers, and the consequential sedentary lifestyle has resulted in children struggling with adult medical problems including obesity, diabetes, and heart disease.

During the last twenty-five years, obesity in children has quadrupled in the United Kingdom. About 27 per cent of children under the age of 11 are overweight, and 13 per cent are obese. In America, the percentage of overweight children ages 6–11 has almost doubled since the early 1980s. From 1984 to 2001, the percentage of overweight preschool children aged 2–5 years has nearly doubled. African and Mexican-American youth are more likely to be overweight than non-Hispanic, Caucasian children and adolescents. There are many known health consequences associated with childhood obesity, which include the following:

- Heart-related problems such as increased blood pressure and cholesterol levels

- Problems with blood sugar and insulin levels, resulting in diabetes

- Mental-health problems such as low self-esteem and depression

- Breathing problems such as asthma and sleep apnoea

- Liver problems such as fatty liver, which results in a type of hepatitis

- Problems with the hip bones
- The risk of obesity persisting into adulthood

While the problem is obvious, the solution doesn't always seem quite so clear. Although the task of raising healthy kids can seem daunting at times, there are fortunately things that even busy parents can do to ensure their children grow up healthy and happy. These include the following:

1. Provide emotional support.

Children need the support and love of family and friends. They need you to respond to both their physical and emotional needs. Find out what is going on with them and how they are making decisions and handling problems. Communicate daily with your children, and regularly discuss with them the importance of making positive choices and resisting dangerous habits, such as smoking, drinking alcohol, or taking drugs. (Even if you had those habits when you were younger, you do have the right – and responsibility – to tell your children to avoid those behaviours.)

Avoid negative comments about their bodies, because that will only contribute to feelings of guilt. Instead, help them set goals towards a healthier lifestyle. Praise them when they participate in active games or eat more vegetables and fewer sweets.

2. Use logic.

Part of helping children take care of themselves is helping them understand why healthy lifestyle is important. In daily encounters, when children ask questions ("What's wrong with eating potato chips?" or "Why do I need to go outside and play?"), it is essential that parents welcome the questions and use those opportunities to logically help kids understand health principles.

3. Do not be child-centered.

Of course, you never want to be insensitive or neglect your child, but the truth is, if you want to raise healthy children, you can't cave in and cater to their every whim and fancy when it comes to food and lifestyle. Instead, help them develop skills to make wise, healthy choices rather than shortsighted, selfish ones. We were designed to enjoy life, and making wise choices will help us do that, "so whether you eat or drink or whatever you do, do it all for the glory of God" (1 Corinthians 10: 31).

4. Be a good role model.

Children watch parents in all areas of life, including their health habits. Only three out of ten young people reported that their parents or other adults actually modelled positive, responsible behaviour, according to the Search Institute (which studies the needs of young people) in their survey of 15,000 American youth in grades 6–12.

Your children need to see you model responsible behaviours. Don't secretly eat snacks or spend lots of time watching television instead of exercising, unless you want your kids to end up doing the same. Remember, teaching is most effective when it is coupled with modelling.

5. Use affirmative discipline.

It is up to parents to set nutritional goals at home. For example, you can establish the rule that family members must eat five servings of fruits and vegetables each day before having a small treat. Don't be afraid to set clear boundaries and have high expectations. Be consistent and firm, but always avoid ridicule and punishment when they make a poor choice. Instead, use encouragement and reasoning to cheer them on when they make good choices.

6. Help children make healthy decisions.

Part of the parent's role is to make children learn how to make safe and healthy choices, such as wearing a seat belt, brushing their teeth, washing their hands, eating nutritious food, and forming healthy relationships. Your approach to teaching decision-making will vary depending on the child's age. For example, with young people, you can start out by offering them a variety of healthy foods and guiding them on how much of each they need to eat. For older children, you can take them grocery shopping and actively involve them. Teach them to read the nutritional ingredients on the labels of their favourite foods. Encourage them to choose foods that are closest to their natural state (thus retaining most of their nutrients), such as baked potatoes instead of chips, fresh apples instead of apple pie, or fresh peas instead of canned peas. For less healthy foods, such as desserts, teach them to exercise moderation.

7. Get physical.

It is an unacceptable fact that many children watch too much TV and don't get enough exercise. To change this pattern, parents can experiment with limiting television, videos, and computer games to less than one hour a day, substituting the rest of the leisure time with outdoor activities. Take walks, ride bicycles, go skateboarding, or play baseball together as a family. Another meaningful and creative way to be active as a family is to find service-oriented activities, such as doing household chores for someone, raking a neighbour's lawn, moving furniture, or cleaning up a community centre. Such projects will teach kids the importance of both activity and service.

8. Do not over schedule.

Music lessons, French class, Little League practice, ballet class – the list of children's ECAs (extracurricular activities) could go on and on – not to mention all the homework. Do these poor kids ever get to play? Keep in mind that healthy development comes from living a balanced life, so don't over schedule your child's life. Remember that what you and your family do today will affect the future. So begin now to invest in a healthy future for your family by exercising regularly, eating well, serving others, and practicing a healthy lifestyle.

Note: It is not just what you eat that packs on the pounds; it is also your pastimes. People who spend more time in front of computers have a higher obesity risk, according to an Australian study. Those individuals with the highest levels of computer use were 1.5 times more likely to be overweight and 2.5 times more likely to be obese than people who don't use computers at all.

The Pursuit of Happiness

A good friend of mine was driving one rainy morning, when his car suddenly hit an oily patch and spun out of control. His attempts to regain control of the vehicle were futile. The car swerved down the road and began to roll. After what seemed like eternity, the car came to a stop, right side up. As he sat clutching the steering wheel in a hot sweat – shaken but uninjured – the radio started playing the song "Don't Worry, Be Happy". Laughable now, the sentiment was a good one at the time, but a little challenging to implement under the circumstances.

The Pursuit

Anne Frank once asserted, "We all live with the objective of being happy; our lives are all different yet the same." Indeed, we are all on a common quest – the pursuit of happiness. So how can we discover it? A good way to start is to identify the things that do *not* guarantee happiness. A common misconception is that money, and plenty of it, is integral to a happy life. Research indicates that in order to be happy we do need the basics. It is certainly more challenging to be cheery when you are sitting in the rain because you do not have a roof over your head, while your tummy screams at you for some filling, but after our basic needs are met, it seems that money contributes little to our level of happiness. It is true: happiness cannot be bought.

Success in a career doesn't guarantee happiness, either. If it is happiness you are seeking, pursuing it by climbing the corporate ladder could find you staring at the wrong wall.

Studies within companies have found similar levels of happiness from the entry-level workers up through senior management. Especially, it is not the type of work we do that promotes or reduces our level of happiness; it is what that work *means* to us that makes the difference.

Finally, even love doesn't promise happiness. Married people report similar levels of happiness to single individuals, except around the dating and wedding times, when there is an upward trend in happiness scores. The peak tends to level out once married life becomes routine, and happiness scores return to baseline. Yet while love does not promise happiness, it may provide the opportunity for it. In one survey, individuals commonly reported that family (especially children) and friends brought them the greatest joy in their lives. Indeed, relationships have the effect of magnifying our emotions – the good get better and the bad get worse. It would seem, then, that if times with family and friends are mostly happy ones, then our lives will be significantly enriched.

If money, career, and relationships are not happiness guarantors, what is the best path to happiness? The answer depends on the type of happiness you are seeking. Pioneer happiness researcher Dr Martin Seligman has identified three levels of happiness.

Level 1: Pleasure

A good giggle does us a world of good. Laughter stimulates the release of stress-relieving hormones similar to those released during strenuous exercise, and so the "high" we get from laughter is a real one.

Undeniably, to laugh is pleasurable, and pleasure makes us happy, but there is a downside. Laughter is not limitless. Pleasure is never permanent. Even the best jokes lose their punch the third or fourth time round, and our most-enjoyed activities wear thin unless there is new twist. So, in the pursuit of happiness, pleasure is problematic. If our happiness is founded in our ability to attain and maintain pleasure, we are destined for discontent. John D. Rockefeller once asserted, "I can think of nothing less pleasurable than a life devoted to pleasure."

This is not to denigrate pleasure, but we should recognize that it is, in fact, a superficial form of happiness. In the Bible, wise King Soloman advised "Take delight in each light-filled hour," but then he added, with a word of caution, "remembering that there will also be many dark days" (Ecclesiastes 11:7–8, "The Message").

Level 2: Engagement

Dr Cheeksentmihi (pronounced "Cheek-sent-me-high") is a world authority on happiness (how could you not be happy with a name like that?). In one study, he issued to individuals pagers that would buzz at random times during the day. When the pager sounded, the individual would document what they were doing and how "into it" they were. He found that when people were engaged in an activity, they experienced "flow", a state in which they were completely engrossed in the experience and felt as if they were truly alive. Not surprisingly, individuals who spent a good portion of their time engaged or absorbed in what they were doing reported higher levels of overall life happiness than those who lived a less-engaged existence.

The take-away message is so simple, it's almost a cliché: *We should do what we love and love what we do.* Spending as much time as we can in a state of flow is a great strategy for boosting our happiness quotient. For this reason, we need to enjoy our work – after all, we do spend almost half of our waking lives at work. Yet, even when we enjoy much pleasure and are regularly engaged in life, we can still find something is lacking. Our happiness may not be complete. To complete the happiness equation, we require a third factor – the deepest level of happiness.

Level 3: Meaning

We all need to feel that our lives have significance and meaning. Studies show that discovering meaning in life will lead to an authentic, steadfast happiness. So from what do we derive meaning?

Discovering meaning in life starts with a conviction that we are of value and have something worthwhile to contribute. It is fostered by knowing that we are a part of something bigger than ourselves and, like an organ of the body, are necessary and needed. An article in *Scientific American Mind* questioned why humans are the only species willing to offer help to complete strangers, even when we have nothing to gain from it. The authors concluded, "Our species is apparently the only one with a genetic make-up that promotes selflessness and altruistic behaviour." Sometimes, deep within, our fabric embraces the paradox that through giving (our talents and our energies) we receive (deep happiness).

Indeed, the pursuit of happiness is incomplete until we make a careful examination of who we are, discover our unique part to play, and then start living it. As a bonus, when we experience meaning (the highest level of happiness), we also will experience the other two levels of happiness: pleasure and engagement. In the words of Katharine Graham, "To love what you do and know it matters – how could anything be more fun?"

The big question is, does God want us to be happy?

TIME magazine ran an article with the intriguing title "Does God Want Us to Be Happy?" Many people doubtlessly view God as a killjoy, so perhaps the question needs to be asked. It may seem surprising, but Jesus showed a great interest in our happiness. Some of His most famous teachings are the Beatitudes, a series of declarations of blessedness. Each declaration begins with the words "Happy are those" (Mathew 5: 3–10) and describes a meaningful way to find happiness, such as being a peacemaker or showing mercy to others. Indeed, these teachings reveal God's desire for us to be happy, but His teachings indicate He was more interested in a life framed by meaning than one punctuated with pleasure. The aim is to be happy, but not selfishly so.

What Makes People Happy?

During a twenty-five-year study of almost 150,000 German adults, a team of scientists from Germany, the Netherlands, and Australia found a strong correlation between the life choices people made and their levels of life satisfaction. The life choices included the following:

Marrying someone with favourable personality traits. The researchers found that neuroticism (a tendency towards emotional instability and anxiety) affects people's happiness the most. Those who married neurotic types were less happy than those who married non-neurotic types.

Valuing family and altruistic goals. People were happier who assigned relatively high value to altruistic goals (such as helping other people and being involved in social and political activities) and family goals (such as having a good marriage and good relationship with children) rather than career goals. Women were also happier when their male partners ranked family goals high.

Church attendance. In this study, the participants who regularly attended church were happier than those who did not. The researchers were unable to ascertain whether it was religious belief or the associated behaviour (such as volunteering, giving and receiving social support, and valuing altruistic and family goals) that affected life satisfaction.

Working as much as you want to. Participants' happiness levels depended on how well they felt their work hours matched their desired work hours. In other words, people who worked more hours or fewer hours than they preferred were less happy. Working less or being unemployed was found to be worse than working too much, presumably because underemployment has financial implications, the researchers wrote.

Social participation and healthy lifestyles. Social interaction and active lifestyles were both associated with happiness of body weight. However, the underweight men and obese women were more likely to be unhappy.

When I was five years old, my mother told me that happiness was the key to life. When I went to school, they asked me what I wanted to be when I grew up. I wrote down "happy". They told me I didn't understand the assignment. I told them they didn't understand life.

Be happy; it is the way to be wise.

(John Lennon)

How Healthy Are You Financially?

How often have you said at the beginning of the new year, "This is the year I am going to follow a budget and put something away in savings. No more procrastinating. This year, for sure, I am resolved to put my finances in order."? Sound familiar? Congratulations – you are not alone. Resolve from now on to avoid the following seven deadly financial flops.

Paying high interest. According to recent research, the average credit card balance an American carries is approximately $10,000. Over 70 per cent of consumers do not pay off their credit card debt in full within the grace period. Save 12–26 per cent interest by eliminating the balance as quickly as possible.

Failing to plan for emergencies. Life events happen unexpectedly: your vehicle breaks down, or your child is rushed to the emergency room. Such events can throw your finances into chaos. Begin saving immediately for an emergency fund, so you can take these emergencies in financial stride. For the average family, a good starting figure is approximately $1,000. Begin this month to save $25–$50 per period until you have that $1,000.

Disregarding savings. Over the last decade, the amount of disposable income the average American has saved each year has been between zero and two per cent. Compare this to other countries, where the average is 10–20 per cent. The most successful way to save is to set a yearly savings goal or to save for a particular project. The best method to do this is to have your employer deduct a set amount per period and send it directly to your bank or credit union. Keep this slogan in mind: what you don't see, you don't miss (and hopefully won't spend).

Omitting that extra principle. Owning a home is the ultimate American and British dream, but don't turn it into a financial nightmare by paying thousands more in interest than you need to. Maybe you should take advantage of current low interest rates and refinance to lower your mortgage payments. Did you know that if you pay an extra $100 in principle per month on a $100,000 home loan, you can save approximately $90,000 in interest over the life of a 30-year mortgage and reduce the time to pay off your mortgage by about eight years? Talk to your banker.

Shunning retirement plans. It is easier to ignore the need to save for retirement when you are establishing your career. One of the best formulas is to set aside 10 per cent of your income if you are in your twenties or thirties; 15–20 per cent if you are in your forties; and if you have failed to save for your future needs, 30 per cent in your fifties to sixties. Most retirement plans give you a tax break on the amount you contribute. For example, you can save $280 per $1,000 invested if you are in the 28 per cent tax bracket. Remember that in the twenty-first century, social security will only provide for approximately 40 per cent of your retirement income.

Neglecting your will. Over 70 per cent of adults do not have a will or a trust. If you die without either of these, the state will dispose of your property and assets and will decide whom your children will reside with – probably not the way you would choose. Call your local conference

Gift Planning & Trust Services department (where wills are usually *free*), or your personal lawyer, or do it yourself on a will-preparation computer program.

Forgetting God. Some of you will say that number seven should have been first, rather than last, on this list – and I agree. I made it number seven so it would be the last item for you to remember. Faithfully paying tithe reminds you that God is the owner and you are His manager. Neglecting local church budget puts all the burden on the other members of your congregation to pay for utilities, education subsidy, Bible materials, etc. Remember to be a cheerful Christian giver.

In the house of the wise are stores of choice food and oil, but a foolish man devours all he has
(Proverbs 21: 20).

Financial Health for Kids: Three Tips for a Great Start

I believe that you are never too young to learn to wisely manage your money. Just imagine if this was a compulsory subject taught in grade school. Would the global financial crisis have been less severe – if not altogether avoided? That wasn't a rhetorical question, friends. In our education system we have a mantra that is continuously drilled into our heads – that we should knuckle down, study hard, and get good grades so that we can find ourselves secure jobs that see us to retirement.

For one thing, the employment landscape has changed so much in the last twenty-five years that if you are 22 years old and reading this, you will very possibly be on to your third job before you are 30. The pace at which technology is changing, and the rate at which business models are evolving, means that you need to revise your thoughts on having only one job for life. So back to the topic at hand: as parents, how do you model to your kids on the issue of money? What you say and do with the money you earn will to a large degree determine how your children deal with their own hard-earned money when they are old enough to do so. Some tips to get them on the right track are as follows:

The 70:20:10 rule. Explain to them that they are allowed to spend 70 cents on anything they want, but 20 cents has to go into the bank. Kids will ask why, and the answer is that it is seed money that they will lend the bank. Explain to them that the bank has to pay them extra (interest) for borrowing their money. It is empowering for your children to know that they are doing the bank a favour, not the other way round.

Tithing: **the other ten cents**. This ten cents teaches your children the idea of giving to charitable causes and creates generosity of spirit. One great way is to discuss with your kids that by tithing they can help people less fortunate than themselves. Explain to them how it makes for a better community when everybody pitches in. It is a fantastic way to build your child's self-esteem.

Delayed gratification. We all want it *now*! Advertisers know how to push the right buttons, but as we have seen, there are a lot of under-25s who are declared bankrupts. They have used the instant credit offered by retailers, for the latest gadgets, only to find that they cannot repay the debt. Personally, I think that having a bad credit rating is as bad as having an STD; no one will want to do business with you, and even worse, one day you may realize that you have the chance to buy into a great business but cannot get financing to do so. If your child desperately wants something now and has money saved, ask him or her to sleep on it for two whole days before going to the store to get it. It is not being cruel to your child but getting him or her to think about wants versus needs. Above all, have open and honest communication with your child about money – it is not a dirty word.

Laughter: How Much Does It Add to Your Health?

Laughter is the best strong medicine for mind and body. It has physical, mental, and social health benefits. The sound of roaring laughter is far more contagious than any cough, sniffle, or sneeze. When laughter is shared, it binds people together and increases happiness and intimacy. In addition to the domino effect of joy and amusement, laughter actually triggers healthy physical changes in the body. Humour and laughter strengthen your immune system, boost your energy, diminish pain, and protect you from the damaging effects of stress. Best of all, this priceless medicine is fun, free, and easy to use.

Have a Laugh: Your Health and Safety

As you carry on with your day-to-day living, think about how well you know your hymns. How well do they communicate to you with regards to your health and safety? The following are just a few thoughts that may make you laugh:

Dentist's hymn: I'll wear a Crown

Weatherman's hymn: Shower of Blessings

Contractor's hymn: I'm Building a Home

The tailor's hymn: Holy, Holy, Holy

The plumber's hymn: There's a Leak in the Old Building

The golfer's hymn: There is a Green Hill Far Away

The politician's hymn: Standing on the Promises

Optometrist's hymn: Open My Eyes That I Might See

The IRS agent's hymn: I Surrender All

The policeman's hymn: Jesus is My Rock, My Sword, and Shield

The gossip's hymn: Pass It On

The single woman's aim: Amen, Amen, Amen

The electrician's hymn: This Little Life of Mine

The florist's hymn: There's a Lily in the Valley

The shopper's hymn: The Sweet By and By

The realtor's hymn: I've Got a New Home Over in Zion

The massage therapists', hymn: He Touched Me

The doctor's hymn: Come on in My Room – Jesus is All My Prescriptions

And for those who speed on the highway, here are a few more hymns:

45 mph: God Will Take Care of You

65 mph: Nearer my God to Thee

85 mph: This World is Not My Home

95 mph: Lord, I'm Coming Home

100 mph: Precious Memories

Note: Life would be so dull without humour and it would be shortened. You would see no reason to live, despite being surrounded by the beauty and diversity given freely by God. Ask God, therefore, to give you a sense of humour and the grace to see a joke. The ability to get humour out of life and pass it on to other people will prolong their lives and yours on this planet earth.

Seek Wisdom to Achieve Health and Wealth

A library of wisdom is more precious than all wealth, and all things that are desirable cannot be compared to it. Whoever therefore claims to be zealous of truth, of happiness, of wisdom or knowledge, must become a lover of books.

(Charles Dickens)

Wisdom is not a product of schooling but of the lifelong attempt to acquire it. Never mistake knowledge for wisdom; one helps you make a living; the other helps you make life.

(Albert Einstein)

For everything you have missed, you have gained something else, and for everything you gain, you lose something else

(Ralph Waldo Emerson)

Wise men speak because they have something to say; fools because they have to say something.

(Plato)

Great minds discuss ideas, average minds discuss events, small minds discuss others.

(Eleanor Roosevelt)

Knowing others is intelligence, knowing yourself is true wisdom. Mastering others is strength; mastering yourself is true power.

(Lao Tzu)

The future belongs to those who believe in the beauty of their dreams.

(Eleanor Roosevelt)

It is better to light a candle than to curse the darkness.

(Chinese proverb often quoted by Eleanor Roosevelt)

Ordinary riches can be stolen, real riches cannot. In your soul are infinitely precious things that cannot be taken from you.

(Oscar Wilde)

Wealth is the product of man's capacity to think.

(Ayn Rand)

Wealth is the ability to fully experience life.

(Henry David Thoreau)

Health is the greatest gift, contentment the greatest wealth, faithfulness the best relationship: Every human being is the author of his own health and disease.

Buddha

The only way to keep your health is to eat what you don't want, drink what you don't like, and do what you'd rather not.

(Mark Twain)

When all is said and done, I know what I have given you, but I don't know what you have received. Remember, the fear of the Lord is the beginning of all wisdom. May you and I seek that wisdom, for healthy and wealthy families and to achieve total well-being. This is all because of the belief that we all have what it takes and we can do all things through Christ who strengthens us.

About the Author

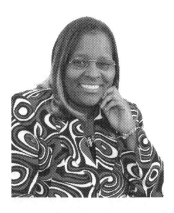

Cecily is known for her very quiet, yet very powerful, ways of inspiring and influencing people for change. She is a strong believer in and an activist for healthier and wealthier families, which form the foundation of a healthier and wealthier society. Cecily is the founder of the dynamic Utulivu organization, which is all about equipping women, men, and youth with powerful strategies and principles to promote purposeful and successful living. She encourages people to thirst for wisdom and seek it through the fear of God and through education.

CMI, BA, BSC, MSC HPPH

Author: *Becoming the Better You*

Dealing with and Overcoming the Challenges of the Twenty-First Century

Founder: Utulivu Organization